A YEAR OF
LIVING
CONSCIOUSLY

A YEAR OF LIVING CONSCIOUSLY

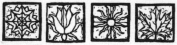

365 DAILY INSPIRATIONS FOR CREATING A LIFE OF PASSION AND PURPOSE

GAY HENDRICKS, PH.D.

WITH RESEARCH AND ADDITIONAL CONTRIBUTIONS BY
LAURA JOYCE, M.A.

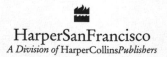

HarperSanFrancisco
A Division of HarperCollins*Publishers*

HarperCollins books may be purchased for educational, business, or sales promotional use. For information please write: Special Markets Department, HarperCollins Publishers, 10 East 53rd Street, New York, NY 10022.

HarperCollins Web Site: http://www.harpercollins.com

HarperCollins®, 📖®, and HarperSanFrancisco™ are trademarks of HarperCollins Publishers, Inc.

FIRST EDITION

Designed by Joseph Rutt

Library of Congress Cataloging-in-Publication Data
Hendricks, Gay.
A year of living consciously : 365 daily inspirations for creating a life of passion and purpose / Gay Hendricks ; with research and additional contributions by Laura Joyce. — 1st ed.
ISBN: 0–06–251588-8 (pbk.)
1. Conduct of Life. 2. Self-realization. 3. Affirmations.
BJ1581.2.H448   1998
1170'.44—dc21   98–30671

99 00 01 02 ❖/RRD 10 9 8 7 6 5 4 3

For Katie
   and for
Christopher, Timothy, and Benjamin

A PERSONAL
INTRODUCTION

A daily guide to a year of living consciously—what a thrilling idea! That was my reaction when a woman came up to me after a lecture some years ago, asking if such a book existed. She said it would be helpful to have a day-at-a-time guide, so that she could learn a bite-sized piece of just-in-time wisdom and meditate on it throughout her day. I told her I wished such a book existed, too, and promised her I would consider writing it someday.

My thirty-second interaction with her led to a three-year process of gathering material and writing the book. In short, I took her hint, and you're holding the result. If the mystery woman whose question inspired the whole enterprise happens to read these words, I invite her to drop me a note and get a generous supply of the book. For me, the concepts and practices in this book are not only the heart of my work but a way of life. I have spent the past thirty years working with people in their journey of conscious living. The wisdom in this book has given me more than a world of pleasure and exhilarating learning—it has given me my life. Nothing between these covers is here simply because it sounds good or looks good. Every idea and practice here has been "kitchen tested" in the rigorous laboratory of real life. In other words, it isn't in this book unless it's helped real people solve real problems.

People have been journeying along the path of conscious living for thousands of years. For a very long time, humans have felt deep urges to discover the truth about how life actually works. Over the centuries, a body of living wisdom has formed, a body we can draw from every moment of our lives. In addition to being a therapist for thirty years—and therefore concerned with helping real people solve real problems—I have also been fascinated with the study of what others have had to say about conscious living over the centuries. Based on my own experience and the study of sources such as Epictetus, Lao-Tzu, William James, and dozens of others, I have come to realize that human beings have been tapping into a fresh-flowing stream of wisdom for at least the past several thousand years.

What does this wisdom have to tell us?

FOUNDATION PREMISES OF CONSCIOUS LIVING

Throughout your year of living consciously, you will see certain themes repeat themselves, just as certain themes repeat themselves in your own life.

Here are some of the foundation ideas on which anyone's journey of conscious living is based. If you open the pages of Epictetus (and I highly recommend that you do), you will see themes similar to the ones we address in this book: self-esteem, relationship, the conscious design of a meaningful life, emotional literacy, and others.

GUIDING PREMISE ONE

Authenticity is essential. A truthful life is both the outcome of the journey and the means of getting there. A successful life is an authentic life. Happiness and creativity rest on a foundation of transparency to yourself and others. Knowing your own heart and speaking clearly to others keep you on the path.

GUIDING PREMISE TWO

Things that can be felt and seen—peace of mind, happiness, and the humane treatment of others—are higher-priority goals than religious concepts such as original sin or beliefs about life after death. The journey of conscious living is based on getting to a deeper level in yourself than beliefs and opinions, in order to experience the essence of what unifies people, not divides them.

GUIDING PREMISE THREE

Conscious living depends on finding out what goals are important to you, and moving toward those goals at a pace that allows you to feel vibrant.

GUIDING PREMISE FOUR

The journey of conscious living begins when you take full responsibility for your life, and slams to a halt when you avoid responsibility for anything.

GUIDING PREMISE FIVE

Happiness, success, and sound relationships depend on letting go of controlling things that are beyond your control. Examples of things you cannot control are the feelings of others, the future, the past, and whether or not other people like you.

GUIDING PREMISE SIX

Spiritual growth comes through a deep embrace of reality, not through flights of arguable fancy. Transcendence is best accomplished by thoroughly acknowledging—rather than ignoring or denying—such human realities as emotions, sexuality, and conflict.

GUIDING PREMISE SEVEN

It is possible to make rapid shifts in consciousness—from scarcity to abundance, from defensiveness to openness, from fear to love—and these shifts in consciousness will change the outer circumstances of your life.

GUIDING PREMISE EIGHT

Peace of mind comes ultimately from making your deepest creative contribution to the community around you. When you make your full contribution, you feel happy, fulfilled, and at ease. When you don't, you don't.

GUIDING PREMISE NINE

Commitment to certain key values—honesty, responsibility, gratitude—not only gives you an inner flow of harmony but also rewards you with an authentic form of power that can be recognized by others. Authentic power comes from authenticity; false power comes from control and ego-aggrandizement.

GUIDING PREMISE TEN

You can choose to become the source of attitudes such as gratitude and responsibility (rather than waiting for the events of life to inspire you to adopt them). If you wait for events to trigger those attitudes, you remain locked in a consumer rather than producer mode, and keep yourself trapped in scarcity.

USING THIS BOOK

As your year of conscious living proceeds, you will notice that these premises and other related themes repeat themselves, each time evolving to a deeper level or revealing a different facet. Think of this year of living consciously as an evolutionary spiral in which you soar in ever-expanding circles. As your consciousness grows upward on the spiral, you touch on each turning a foundation theme that you can master at a higher level.

As I began working on this book, I turned to the assistance of a fine writer and insightful therapist who also happens to be my niece and research associate. Laura Joyce, whose voice you will come across from time to time in the book, adds a fresh perspective because she's in a different stage of the life journey than I am. My kids are grown, for example, while hers are running and toddling around the room as she writes (I know this because I often hear them in the background when we talk on the phone). Her input was most valuable.

GOING FORTH

None of us invents the journey of conscious living; we are heir to it. For thousands of years, people from east to west have been looking to the heavens and looking into their own hearts, wondering about the same fundamental questions:

- Who am I?
- Where do I want to go?
- What is my plan for getting there?
- How can I give and receive love to my full potential?
- What is my creative gift and how can I express it?

We are still asking these questions today, and we will no doubt be asking them thousands of years from now. I invite you to join this heartful and mindful community of seekers by making a commitment to a year of living consciously. May your journey be blessed.

JANUARY

The journey of a thousand miles begins with a single step.

BEGINNING THE PATH OF CONSCIOUS LIVING

The journey of living consciously begins with a single moment of commitment, saying yes to the impulse within you that wants to grow, to expand, to embrace your largest possible self, to make your largest possible contribution to the world.

Saying yes does not mean you know how to handle each moment of the journey—and it certainly does not mean you (or anyone else) know how the journey will turn out. What you do when you say yes to the desire to live a more conscious life is to create a field of possibility around you and within you. As a child, my obesity was a problem my family tried to help me with—from special diets to experimental growth-hormone injections. I found myself in my twenties still struggling with the same problem. One magic day I realized I had never made my own commitment to having a healthy body, so I took a vow to get the weight off—no matter what it took. Within a month, I'd lost almost thirty pounds, with seventy more coming off over the next year. It was never easy, but it had never even been possible before. Now, twenty-five years later—6'1" and 190 rather than 6'1" and 320, where I started—I'm more sure than ever that it was that first step that did it. This field of possibility, opened by thousands of people for thousands of years, often has the effect of making life seem richer and more exciting, but always know that the field was opened by your willingness to take that first step.

■ A CONSCIOUS LIVING PRACTICE FOR TODAY ■

On New Year's Eve or New Year's Day, many of you make resolutions. You vow to lose that extra ten pounds, to start exercising, to save more money. I want to urge you to do those things that you know are necessary or worthwhile for you, but here, now, I am urging you to make a different kind of resolution. It is one that some might say is completely without merit, but I know better. Today, I urge you toward the following resolution: *This year, I commit to living consciously, and I commit to having fun as I do. I commit to expanding my consciousness and my capacity for fun every minute of this year.*

....

JANUARY 2

Learning something new is the bestest thing in the world.
—ANDREW HARPER, AGE SEVEN

WHAT CAN I LEARN TODAY?

Think of your journey of conscious living as a learning project, not as a healing project. A learning paradigm offers certain advantages over a therapy or healing paradigm. In the healing and therapy paradigms, you have to think there's something wrong with you before you can get better. In counseling people over the past thirty years, I've watched people struggle with receiving feedback, both from others and from the experiences in their lives. The big problem is that you flip into thinking "What's wrong with me?" when you get some feedback, and then you get defensive or start feeling bad about yourself. In the end, you don't get the message. A learning paradigm does not presume anything is wrong with you; it says simply that there are things you can learn to make your life and work more easeful and productive. In addition, the therapy paradigm often focuses on past events, presumably so a more positive present can be attained. While this may occur, the therapy paradigm often keeps people in thrall to the past, perceiving themselves as victims. The learning paradigm invites you to take full responsibility for your life, to make commitments in the present, to practice those commitments, and to identify goals for the future. The act of doing these things may pull past events to the surface, but they will emerge in the context of a forward-looking journey to the future, not in reference to the past.

■ A CONSCIOUS LIVING PRACTICE FOR TODAY ■

As you go through your activities today, return often to the question "What do I most need to learn right now?"

Realize that your journey is not about being right or achieving anything; it is always about learning what most needs to be learned.

....

JANUARY 3

All the best responsibility is taken.—ANONYMOUS

THE POWER OF HEALTHY RESPONSIBILITY

You all have seen and felt the unpleasant power of unhealthy responsibility. When a martyr takes on the burden of someone else's responsibility, that's unhealthy. And when a blamer places responsibility on somebody else's shoulders, that's unhealthy. The journey of conscious living is a journey of getting the responsibility formula just right: 100 percent for you and 100 percent for me.

Healthy responsibility is defined as taking 100 percent responsibility for yourself while inspiring others to take 100 percent responsibility. Healthy responsibility can be contrasted with two forms of unhealthy responsibility—the condition of less than 100 percent (perceiving yourself as a victim) and the condition of more than 100 percent (perceiving others as victims and you as their caretaker).

■ A CONSCIOUS LIVING PRACTICE FOR TODAY ■

Today, mount a vigilant search for any ways in which you are thinking of yourself as a victim or thinking of others as victims. Begin your inquiry by saying these statements out loud, trying them on like you'd try on a new wardrobe:

- I know how to make clear agreements with others.
- I enter into agreements initiated by others clearly and consciously.
- I can be counted on to do what I say I will do.
- I can be counted on not to do what I say I will not do.
- I know how to handle instances when I break agreements.
- I know how to handle instances when others break agreements with me.
- I know how to change agreements that are not working.
- Others keep their agreements with me.
- I take healthy responsibility for my life and the projects in which I'm involved.

....

JANUARY 4

Grow up, and that is a terribly hard thing to do. It is much easier to skip it and go from one childhood to another.—F. SCOTT FITZGERALD

HOW TO KNOW WHAT YOU'RE COMMITTED TO

It is simple to find out what you're committed to—just look at the results you're creating. A friend was complaining to me that he'd spent a great deal of time and energy hassling with the IRS during the past year. I asked, "Why do you suppose you're so committed to spending your time that way?" "But I'm not committed to that," he began to argue. Then a sheepish smile came over his face as he got the point. Later he phoned with this insight: "If I use my energy fighting the IRS, I don't have to do the tough work of creating some new income streams." Many of you are gripped by the loony idea that your intentions are different from the results you create. It simplifies life enormously the moment you accept that the results you create are your unconscious intentions made visibly manifest.

■ A CONSCIOUS LIVING PRACTICE FOR TODAY ■

Select a particular issue that's troubling you. For example, you might select "squabbling with my spouse all the time." Claim the unconscious intention to create that result: "I squabble with my spouse because I'm committed to squabbling with my spouse all the time." Notice your mind and body wanting to argue with this powerful assertion. But also notice the feeling of exhilaration when you finally own your unconscious intention. You're in the driver's seat.

....

JANUARY 5

There is a period of life when we swallow a knowledge of ourselves and it becomes either good or sour.—PEARL BAILEY

THE NEED TO CHANGE

It is a natural human instinct to focus only briefly on that which needs changing and then to leap precipitously into action. Slow yourself; *stop*. Give yourself the luxury of the thought of letting go before requiring yourself to be practical, gathering your road maps to reckon with what lies ahead. Today is the time for developing your sight, for learning new ways of looking deep within and letting the layers of yourself be revealed in all of their gradual depth and glory. The process is all you have; the end point is of little consequence if you are not present for the journey. Let go of your need to move toward a set end point, to abandon things, to embrace the unfamiliar; there is time for sweeping change later. For today, your work is to peel back a layer of memory, an experience or feeling that has laid itself on your heart. Feel the newness of the self that is still tender underneath. Let it breathe. Love the layer you are uncovering and love yourself for your many facets and layers, especially the ones that have been most hidden within you.

■ A CONSCIOUS LIVING PRACTICE FOR TODAY ■

Find a time when you can be uninterrupted for five to ten minutes. As you immerse yourself in memory, filter out the thoughts that take you away from memory, and lead yourself gently back to this: Remember a time when you have fled some part of yourself precipitously. What were you running from? Why?

As you allow your mind to wander through the memory, embrace and accept all of the feelings as they come: sadness, frustration, anger, shame, fear . . . these feelings are as much a part of you as your strong jaw, your brown eyes, your reddened, glowing skin when you stand in the wind. You might as easily try to recreate your jaw, hide your eyes, forever turn your face from the elements as deny your own feelings. You *are* your feelings, and your feelings are you.

....

JANUARY 6

It seems so natural and easy now to love myself.
How did I ever make it so hard?

NATURAL AND EASY

Those "safe," protected places you create around your heart—the ones designed so that no can hurt you—have one fatal flaw: if no one can hurt you, no one can touch you, either. In the real world of conscious relationships, no one and everyone is safe. The paradox? In a conscious, committed, and honest relationship, you put your heart out into the thick tangle of the truth, and the possibility certainly exists that your heart may end up bruised and battered. A friend who is a hospice worker gave me a powerful example of this point: in sitting with more than a hundred people as they died, she said she'd not even once heard a dying person talk about love not received ... but dozens of her patients had expressed regret about love not given. So, while you may— and, in fact, you are likely to—sometimes experience pain as the result of your new connectedness, you will also have the opportunity time and again to experience soaring joy and a degree of good feeling that may well seem unimaginable to the person with the hiding heart.

■ A CONSCIOUS LIVING PRACTICE FOR TODAY ■

Imagine your secrets and your untruths as something dark, and your truth as light and sun-filled, airy and clean. Close your eyes and breathe. As you exhale slowly, breathe out the dark secrets and untruths that clog the pores of your body; as you slowly and deeply inhale, breathe in the pure, light truth that is yours. Feel the sensations in your body as you breathe and allow a sense of lightness and good feeling to take you over, telling you that you are at peace with and centered in truth. Return yourself to the physicality of good feeling by focusing on these feelings when you feel yourself wandering from the conscious path.

....

JANUARY 7

I think that we may safely trust a good deal more than we do.
—HENRY DAVID THOREAU

THE OVER-RIPE HEART

A pseudo-safety is created when you put your heart in hiding. It's natural for any creature to cringe and go into contraction when wounded, but the courageous human must unfold from the contraction and risk again in order to grow. After a painful breakup with my first love, I kept my heart sealed off for years. Looking back on it, I don't think I learned one useful thing about relationships in that whole time of hiding myself. Finally, I came out of hiding and into the world again. Sure enough, while I've felt my share of pain while out here in the living world, I have also felt once again the exhilaration of growth.

■ A CONSCIOUS LIVING PRACTICE FOR TODAY ■

Ask yourself several key questions today:

- What am I hiding?
- What or who am I hiding from?
- What is the payoff for hiding?
- What is the cost of hiding?

....

JANUARY 8

Nothing is so burdensome as a secret.——FRENCH PROVERB

SECRETS

What is your greatest secret, the thing you have thought, felt, or done that you hold closest to the vest? Think on it for a moment and consider why you have relegated it to the hiding place of your heart. If shame keeps your secret where it is, recognize that your heart will be like a petri dish, and your shame the darkness and dampness that allow disease to flourish, to grow from something small and contained into something that can take on a virulent life of its own. The only way to cleanse yourself is to open your heart up to the air. A married couple told me a simple yet remarkable story: They were playing a card game together one evening when he did something that irritated her. She didn't say anything about it, and a few minutes later, she noticed a red band of irritation under her wedding ring. It seemed to have come from nowhere. She had recently heard a lecture on the mind/body connection, and it occurred to her that the unspoken communication with her husband was expressing itself through the rash on her finger. She took a deep breath and told her husband what she was irritated about. Within a few minutes, the rash was completely gone. Secrets do not flourish in the light, and they do not take you over if you do not allow yourself to be at their mercy. Take ownership of your secret; take it on with the knowledge that you are bigger than any secret you might hold dear. It cannot own you or control you without your acquiescence.

■ A CONSCIOUS LIVING PRACTICE FOR TODAY ■

Find a light, quiet place and time so that you will not be disturbed. With a pen and paper, write down your secret in as few words as possible and focus on what you have written. Breathe deeply, feeling the clean, fresh air as it flows through you. Put down the paper on which you have written your secret; recognize this moment as the one in which you have separated yourself from the darkness of the secret that has been inside of you. It is now outside of you, and what is inside still needs loving acceptance and healing, but you have begun the process today.

....

JANUARY 9

All human unhappiness comes from not facing reality squarely, exactly as it is.
—BUDDHA

ELIMINATING UNNECESSARY TENSION

The journey of living consciously gets smoother the moment you learn a simple principle, one that may take a lifetime to master. The principle is this: Stress and tension are caused not by the events of life itself but by avoiding four required responses to the events. The more you avoid the four required responses, the more tension builds up, not only in your body but in the body of organizations, too. Tension builds first when you don't face or accept the reality of a situation. The key to effective action is to accept things first exactly as they are. Tension continues to build when you avoid making choices, and reaches its peak when you avoid taking action. For example, if you have a relationship conflict, tension will build until you make two key moves, facing and accepting that there is a problem. Once that has been faced and accepted, you can choose a path of action and make appropriate steps. Few of you would drive a car with a flat back tire for months or years—the tension would drive you to distraction. Unfortunately, I have seen people avoid facing a problem for years, a problem that could have been faced and dealt with in a matter of minutes.

■ A CONSCIOUS LIVING PRACTICE FOR TODAY ■

Take a moment today to ask yourself a key question: "Is there anything in my life I'm avoiding facing and accepting?" If you think of something, pause and deal with it directly. Take a moment now to accept it, just as it is.

....

JANUARY 10

I don't give them hell. I just tell the truth and they think it is hell.—HARRY S. TRUMAN

JOY AND LAUGHTER

What if, instead of unearthing pain and buried hurts and anxieties when you take your first steps down the path toward conscious living, you find joy and laughter? Are you someone who knows in your gut that relationship is supposed to be difficult—hard work, hard communication, hard thought, hard feeling? Consider another alternative: although there's focused work involved, living and loving consciously is pure, exuberant fun! I have seen many couples laughing and holding hands moments after telling some long-withheld truth, something they'd feared speaking to each other about for weeks or months.

In letting feelings up to breathe the air, you put a stop to the dark, difficult, cloak-and-dagger existence that speaks of shame. Instead, you turn your face upward toward the sun in a celebration of self-pride.

■ A CONSCIOUS LIVING PRACTICE FOR TODAY ■

It is your turn to practice telling the truth about that which is unarguable: who you are and how you feel. Today, ask yourself how you are. Make a deep and honest and intentional inquiry into your heart and mind; allow your mind to play over your physical and emotional being and take stock of where you stand. When your partner or a close friend asks you how you are today, your answer will be ready to spring from your heart, no longer suppressed or covered with the brittle veneer of acceptability. Instead, your irrepressible self will shine through.

Try saying how you feel today.

Some possible feelings (every one of them your truth, your facts): happy . . . lonely . . . confused . . . satisfied . . . angry . . . excited . . .

....

JANUARY 11

I often marvel how it is that though each man loves himself beyond all else, he should yet value his own opinion of himself less than that of others.—MARCUS AURELIUS

MY COMMITMENT TO POTENTIAL

How did you end up sitting here, in this chair, on this day, reading these words? Some firm or tremulous voice—perhaps both—has made its call to you and brought you here, up from the gray unconscious and into the light that is conscious living. You have the faith and the courage to let yourself listen. The voice is your voice, your heart that is open and crying out for change. Here is the first truth you can tell yourself: *I am here today because my commitment to living my potential is greater than my commitment to the familiar.* I want to be alive. I want to scald myself on burning truths and heal myself with soothing, cool honesty. I want things that I may have been told were too much to expect, but I put my foot down here and now. Breathing room for my essence—integrity, in other words— is not too much to demand; it is my due.

■ A CONSCIOUS LIVING PRACTICE FOR TODAY ■

Throughout the day, take frequent ten-second breaks to recognize the journey you have undertaken, and to affirm yourself for being open to the journey.

Affirmation: *Today I make a commitment to learning and growing that is bigger than my commitment to staying the same.*

Remember to breathe deeply before, during, and after your affirmation. You are cleansing both your mind and the very fibers of your body as you breathe deeply and simultaneously affirm yourself.

Return to this affirmation throughout the day, particularly when you feel tension or anxiety arising from everyday interactions. Harness the energy wasted on low-dividend emotions such as frustration, and channel it into positive, affirming energy.

Remind yourself: I am here today for the good of my heart.

....

JANUARY 12

No man can reveal to you aught but that which already lies half asleep in the dawning of your knowledge.—KAHLIL GIBRAN

HONORING YOUR ROOTS

Honor your roots of the past, the truths and experiences that form your history—that about you that is rooted deep in the heart of life.

Honor your branches, the dancing, breathing, living testimony to your openness to growth and change. Even though you may wish to let go of parts of you, especially parts of your past, the only things to be released are behaviors; your history and memories cannot be released. They are *in* you and *of* you as certainly as your heart, and you would be wise to recognize their permanence. This is not to say that you must allow your past to rule you. Instead, you must learn to be ever vigilant in order to honor your past and yet keep it from being your present or determining your future. For example, many people struggle in relationship with their parents. In working through my own parental issues, and in helping many others do the same, I have learned that what heals me is to honor my feelings about my parents—whether deep pain or deep gratitude—at the same time that I honor my parents themselves, just as they are. By doing so, I nourish the deep roots of myself and the roots of those who have nourished me.

■ A CONSCIOUS LIVING PRACTICE FOR TODAY ■

What is in you, like the willow tree, that is you and cannot be lived without?

Think of one word that you often use to describe yourself.

Say the word out loud, letting yourself hear it, feel it—know what it means to you. Embrace the word as you say it and as you let yourself know it. Accept your powerful nature, your stability; embrace the part of you that stands tall and unmoved by the winds of change—and embrace with equal acceptance the part of you that sways in the breeze and leans toward the sun, seeking the growth and change that the motion and warmth are sure to bring.

Mr. Dufy lived a short distance from his body.—JAMES JOYCE

EVERY COMMITMENT INVITES A CHALLENGE

Just after you make a big commitment, expect a big challenge to come along. Think of it as the universe's way of making sure you mean business. I made a big commitment to my health some years ago and embarked on a major diet. In the first week I lost five pounds and was beginning to feel better than I had in a long time. Lo and behold, a friend dropped by with a huge box of chocolates. I could actually feel the tug-of-war in my body between my commitment to health and my aching desire for a big chewy caramel. The caramel won that first round, but it made me feel sick, causing me to up my commitment to my well-being.

What you do to get in your own way is more powerful than any obstacle others can place in your path. When inner demons arise, know that they do so because of your commitment to a new way of being. When you make a big commitment, all your inner barriers to it are pushed to the surface to be purified by your acceptance.

■ A CONSCIOUS LIVING PRACTICE FOR TODAY ■

Tune in to the physical sensations you experience when you think about making a soul-level commitment to conscious living. Notice if you feel fear, anger, sadness, or some other sensation or feeling. Accept whatever arises, knowing that it is part of you that wants and needs acceptance.

For all men have one entrance into life . . . —THE APOCRYPHA

REBIRTH

For years I have worked with individuals who had issues dating back to birth, and even to the prenatal stage of life. A birth or pre-birth trauma can color your experience throughout life unless it is brought to consciousness and dealt with lovingly and acceptingly. There are literal manifestations of birth trauma; for instance, someone who was trapped in the birth canal, with panic swirling around the mother just beyond his reach, might experience claustrophobia. Someone else may have a more figurative manifestation of birth trauma; an unwanted child may struggle moment by moment through her life to trust that another truly loves and cherishes her.

For Christians, Easter represents a rebirth—the day that Christ returned to the living, having been allowed to raise himself up from his grave. For non-Christians, this concept may seem odd or questionable. Whatever your beliefs, however, on this day, as many people celebrate a second chance, you can celebrate the same—a second chance to be humbled by your own humanity, by the opportunity and grace that allow you to be imperfect and still loved and loving.

■ A CONSCIOUS LIVING PRACTICE FOR TODAY ■

Take yourself back to the moment of your birth. Imagine the darkness and then the flooding light; the peaceful, rhythmic sounds of the womb and then the loud, living sounds that greeted you upon your birth. Breathe slowly and deeply as you allow yourself to be reborn. Today, your birth is a cause for only celebration, for only love and warmth and acceptance and joy. There are no questions at your birth, no ambivalence, only joyful celebration. You are right to be born, and you have a right to be born. Know this today.

I have no desire to prove anything by dancing . . . I just dance.—FRED ASTAIRE

MAGICAL VEHICLES

Your body is a magical vehicle that carries your experiences, your feelings, your essence. The farther away you are from knowing your body, the farther you move from your essence; the two are inextricably attached. Think about drugs or alcohol as a way that people separate themselves physically from their emotional being. By numbing your body, you numb those feelings clamoring for attention. It is a vicious cycle from which there is only one escape: knowing and embracing and loving yourself, facing yourself head-on without the screen of deception between you and your essence.

A good friend told me about a moment that changed him forever. He had been a dangerously out-of-control alcoholic for sixteen years when a two-minute conversation turned his life rightside up. A therapist pointed out to him that his drinking seemed to be an attempt to drown out one specific feeling, a gnawing loneliness. The therapist said he would eventually have to either let himself feel it—or die. He decided to live, and although he had to confront an ancient demon of a feeling, it passed after a few months (and he hasn't had a drink since that fateful day).

■ A CONSCIOUS LIVING PRACTICE FOR TODAY ■

Close your eyes and let your awareness turn inward. Notice any inner experiences as you take three relaxed, full breaths. Move in a way that expresses the joyfulness of knowing yourself, of being centered. Perhaps you will sway, or perhaps you will dance. Let the movement come to you; let the movement be of you, from you. Open your eyes gently and make three observations, without judgment, of the physical experience of moving in a way that both captured your essence and let it soar.

- My body felt _____.
- I was most aware of my _____.
- That part of me felt _____.

Throughout the day today, be aware of your body: Let yourself feel sensation and movement and connect your emotional experience to your physical one. Perhaps you hold your strongest feelings in your shoulders, your neck, your belly. As you locate the place where your feelings take hold, and as you connect these feelings to your physical self, let this new knowledge serve as a reminder, as a cue that you hold some essential truth inside. Let it out and feel the miraculous change that takes place in your body.

....

JANUARY 16

I have an everyday religion that works for me.
Love yourself first, and everything else falls into line.—LUCILLE BALL

LOVING YOURSELF IS YOUR BIGGEST GIFT TO OTHERS

On the surface it might sound like loving yourself is a selfish act, but it is actually the ultimate act of selfless giving. Egotism and bragging, for example, are so painful to behold because they are signs of self-hatred, not self-love. They are desperate attempts to call attention to yourself after you've sunk into self-loathing. One moment of genuine self-love can result in a lifetime of compassionate contribution to others. One of my friends, a yoga teacher and single parent with several children, told me, "If I take a few minutes in meditation each day to resonate with myself, I can do things all day with and for my kids. But if I don't take a little time for me each day, I end up feeling resentful about all the demands they make."

We could all take a hint from her discovery. Many times in my own life I have gotten mired in relationship conflicts only to realize after a while that the conflict had nothing to do with the other person. When you love the unlovable parts of yourself—anger, fear, grief, or whatever else—the problem with the other person clears up.

■ A CONSCIOUS LIVING PRACTICE FOR TODAY ■

Take five or ten minutes to yourself today. Don't do anything—just sit and be. Appreciate yourself for simply being you. Realize: If I don't take wonderful care of myself, who will?

....

JANUARY 17

If you cannot find it in your own body, where will you wander in search of it?
—THE UPANISHADS

YOUR LIVING BODY OF WISDOM

You may marvel at the Taj Mahal or the Great Pyramids, but every day you walk around in a miracle—your own body—that makes those stone wonders pale by comparison. Your body is a wealth of wisdom and a genuine source of enlightenment . . . when you remember to listen to it. Yet the tendency is to focus on the things that are wrong with your body and to forget to appreciate it for the miracle it is. This is like visiting the Pyramids and focusing on missing chips. Your mind soaks up images all day long, from billboards, television, and magazines. During the course of only one day you may be exposed to several hundred food advertisements without even realizing it. This bombardment of images can make it difficult to listen to your body, to find out, for example, what your body really wants to eat. By the end of a typical day, you may have spent ten steady minutes having images beamed into your head. At least spend the equivalent amount of time listening to your body.

Take a moment right now to honor your body. Give it a moment of silent appreciation for all these years of service.

Ask your body, "What could I do for you today to show I love you?"

....

JANUARY 18

Boldness has genius, power, magic in it.—GOETHE

THE BOLD STEP OF COMMITMENT

Conscious commitment begins the process of positive change. For example, many people had thought about the civil rights movement in the South, but Martin Luther King made a conscious commitment to it. Then, change happened. Many people had thought about going to the moon, but John F. Kennedy made a conscious commitment to getting someone there, feet bouncing on the rocky ground. Once the commitment was made, change happened. I have watched this work on levels both small and grand on a more personal level, as my students and friends have made intentions in life—and have then made those intentions flower and take root.

In your journey of conscious living, begin by making commitments to yourself. Then, change happens.

■ A CONSCIOUS LIVING PRACTICE FOR TODAY ■

Take a few moments in front of the mirror to say these commitments out loud:

- First, commit to self-knowledge: I commit to knowing myself authentically and completely.
- Then, commit to speaking the truth: I commit to expressing myself authentically.

- Third, take a stand for integrity: I commit to acknowledging my feelings, taking responsibility for all my actions, and keeping all my agreements.
- Finally, take a stand for your creativity: I commit to the full embrace and expression of my creativity, and to being a catalyst for the creativity of others.

....

JANUARY 19

What we need are more people who specialize in the impossible.—THEODORE ROETHKE

LIVING IN THE ZONE

In life there are three zones in which learnings occur. Zone One is what you know you know. An example: You know how to drive and you know you know it. Then there's Zone Two, what you know you don't know. An example: You don't know the quadratic equation, and you know you don't know it. However, the key learnings of life usually occur in Zone Three, what you don't know you don't know. An example: Early in my marriage I received feedback that I was emotionally distant. At first I became defensive and denied it. Then I justified it for a while, thinking my wife and others gave me that feedback because they were dependent and clingy. They only thought I was distant because they were envious of my self-reliance! Finally, I had a Zone Three learning that changed my life: I realized that I didn't allow myself to get close to other people because I was afraid that if I did, they would abandon me. If I could keep them a little distant, it wouldn't hurt as much if they left me. My early history had an abandonment element to it, which is likely where I picked up this program. The point is, I hadn't known why I was distant, and I hadn't known that I didn't know it.

Open the power of Zone Three with a conscious commitment. Say out loud, "Today I take a stand of openness to learning whatever I most need to learn. I let go of my expectations that life show up a certain way for me—I take it as it comes, and learn from it as much as I can."

....

JANUARY 20

Man partly is and wholly hopes to be.——ROBERT BROWNING

DEFENDING AGAINST DEFENSIVENESS

Defensiveness is one of the biggest barriers on the path of conscious living. Every time you say, "Wait a minute! This isn't the experience I'm supposed to be having!" you put the brakes on the learning possibilities in that moment. It takes genuine courage to come up against your defensive patterns, then to choose to let them go, making yourself vulnerable. Become familiar with some of the major defensive patterns:

DISTRACTIONS
Q: What are you feeling right now?
A: Let me catch this phone call first, then we can talk.

HOSTILITY
Q: What are you feeling right now?
A: Why are you people always so obsessed with feelings? Whatever happened to good old-fashioned thinking?

OVERINTELLECTUALIZING
Q: What are you feeling right now?
A: My friend Sid said he read a book that said feelings were made up of three chemicals, but I can't remember exactly which they were right now.

TRYING TO PLEASE/APPROVAL-SEEKING
Q: What are you feeling right now?
A: I guess I must be scared—does that sound right to you?

■ A CONSCIOUS LIVING PRACTICE FOR TODAY ■

Today, notice any times you start to feel uncomfortable. At these times, ask yourself what you are defending against right now. When you can catch yourself in the act of going defensive—and then choose to let go of your defensive posture—you can make great leaps ahead on the path of conscious living.

....

JANUARY 21
It is only with the heart that one can see rightly; what is essential is invisible to the eye.
—ANTOINE DE SAINT-EXUPÉRY

MESSAGE SOURCES

If you're feeling or hearing a rattle in your body, it means you haven't committed yourself deeply enough to the path you're traveling. Listen to the sounds of your body—the tension of your muscles, the hesitance or freedom of your breathing, the movement of energy in your wholeness. When I make a big commitment, I often feel a tightening and a quiver of "butterflies" in my stomach. These sensations let me know I'm afraid, which in turn lets me know it's time to make a more thorough commitment. When I made the commitment to embarking on the three-year program for my doctorate, for example, I had those tight, quivery sensations for close to a month. When I finally committed in my body and soul—"Nothing's going to stop me"—the fear sensations disappeared in an instant. Think of fear as a test of commitment, a way to focus your attention on the question, "Is this what I really want?"

State aloud your commitment to conscious living. Use any words you choose. As you say the words out loud, notice if any feelings emerge in your body awareness. Use them as inspirations to deepen your commitment, not as reasons to abandon it.

....

JANUARY 22

If heaven made him, earth can find some use for him.—CHINESE PROVERB

CONSCIOUS LISTENING

One of the most powerful things you can do on any day is to listen consciously. Begin by examining the intentions behind your listening. Some people listen to find fault with what the speaker is saying. Others listen with a "What's in it for me?" intention, while many listen to rebut, argue, or debate. Conscious listening is based on a different set of intentions. Your first intention is to make sure you understand exactly what the other person is saying. Call this "listening for accuracy." A second intention is to resonate with the emotion, if any, under the words. Call this intention "listening for feeling." If the person is angry, for example, your best move is to resonate with the emotion and draw it out so you can understand it. People deeply want to be heard. Seldom do they want advice or opinions or debate. Imagine a world in which people actually listened to each other! To help create such a world, pause often throughout the day to do the following practice.

■ A CONSCIOUS LIVING PRACTICE FOR TODAY ■

When people speak to you today, make a concerted effort to listen for accuracy and emotion. Use phrases like "If I understand you correctly, you're saying _____" and "It sounds like you felt _____ (hurt or sad or angry, for instance)." Avoid giving opinions and advice—instead, see if you can listen so intently that people bring forth their own wisdom.

....

JANUARY 23

Truth always originates in a minority of one.—WILL DURANT

COMMITMENT

I commit to revealing rather than concealing.

I often say that failing to keep an agreement plus telling a dang good story does not equal *keeping* an agreement, and yet look how frequently humans do that very thing, as if we are more clever than the person we are trying to fool—the self. That can't be! If you are clever enough to come up with the lie to cover the commitment that hasn't been honored, you're clever enough to catch yourself in the lie. *Listen to your body.*

Why not short-circuit the whole messy business of self-delusion and take the straight, clear, clean path of truth-telling? Finding your way down the path is more simple than you may think. Take the step of listening to yourself—to the rattles of deception or to the soothing, whispering winds of truth—and you're on your way home.

■ A CONSCIOUS LIVING PRACTICE FOR TODAY ■

Think back on an instance when you wanted to share a secret about yourself with your partner but did not do so. Perhaps at the time you told yourself that you were protecting your partner from the truth. Now it is time to tell *yourself* the truth: The one you were protecting was you, no one else. Walk yourself back through the memory, imagining the outcome if you had told the truth.

When you find yourself in a similar conflict again, cut to the core of why you hide yourself, and prepare for the whole truth. In the world of relationship, lies and secrets are self-defense strategies rather than kindnesses to others, and in the end they always result in distance and entanglement.

....

JANUARY 24

Energy is the only life and is from the Body, and Reason is the bound or outward circumference of Energy.—WILLIAM BLAKE, *THE MARRIAGE OF HEAVEN AND HELL*

AT THE LEVEL OF THE SOUL

The way to get started on the path of the conscious heart is to make a commitment at the level of the soul. It must be something you really want, and you must find your pockets of resistance and deal with them. On your journey to the center of your heart, you make a conscious decision to hold nothing back. Visualize this as the alcoholic who professes a desire to quit drinking but keeps a bottle stashed somewhere, just in case. You must make this special commitment at your very core if you are to arrive safely at the goal: the transformation of yourself intrapersonally and interpersonally. A theory will not change you or rediscover you. Only commitment will, but it must be deep and focused and intentional.

■ A CONSCIOUS LIVING PRACTICE FOR TODAY ■

Ask yourself, "What keeps me from journeying on the path of the conscious heart?"

When you can move quickly from the frozen wasteland of emotional distance to the warmth of a loving embrace, that's a miracle.

My religion is very simple—my religion is kindness.—THE DALAI LAMA

TO THY SELF BE . . . KIND

The first place to mount a campaign of kindness is inside your own mind and heart. Many of you treat yourself with such criticism and contempt that it is hardly surprising that it spills over onto others. Laura writes: I remember a night spent working on homework with my son not so long ago. He was having trouble in school, and his math struggles mirrored ones I'd had when I was around his age. As he struggled to do the work, I heard him mutter, "I'm so stupid." I felt as if I'd been punched in the belly, hearing my own child, the heart of my heart, speak of himself so contemptuously. My gut response was to argue with him ("No, you're not!!") and move on with the assignment, but I caught myself. Instead, we put the work aside for a few moments and I shared my own early math struggles with him, and then we talked about how to love ourselves when we feel least lovable.

Begin a kindness campaign today, starting with your body. Ask yourself: How could I be kind to my body today? Then extend your campaign to your emotions: How could I be kind to my feelings today? Finally, go beyond your own skin with the question: If my religion were kindness, how could I practice my religion with others today?

■ A CONSCIOUS LIVING PRACTICE FOR TODAY ■

Pause ten seconds right now and sense how kindness feels inside you. What does it feel like to be kind? Now picture someone with whom you are likely to interact today. While thinking of that person, imagine surrounding him or her with kindness. Imagine beaming kindness at that person.

If you have time, call to mind several other people with whom you're likely to come into contact today. Surround them with kindness. Then find out what happens when you see them in person.

....

JANUARY 26
A man must make his opportunity, as oft as find it.—Francis Bacon

COMMITTING TO COMMITMENT

Before you can make a specific commitment about truth or responsibility or relationship, you must commit to being committed. This commitment means making a vow to yourself, a vow to wonder, to question, and to come to know your truth without burdening yourself with the limits of judgment and blame.

Both Laura and I have an "inner fat child," the chubby shadow of our former physical selves. We have both observed that it wasn't until we were able to lovingly receive that damaged, unloved child inside of us that we were able to access the healthy, newer physical selves we have fashioned. The receiving began with wondering, Who is this child I feel living sadly inside of me? And the wondering was without judgment: How can I love this child? How can I let this child know he is safe, she is loved?

■ A CONSCIOUS LIVING PRACTICE FOR TODAY ■

Continue to ask yourself about your commitment:

- What is a soul-level commitment and how might I feel having made one?
- How might I phrase a commitment to setting off on this journey and to owning and loving my essence?

JANUARY 27

The first peace, which is the most important, is that which comes within the souls of people when they realize their relationship, their oneness, with the universe and all its powers, and when they realize at the center of the universe dwells the Great Spirit, and that this center is really everywhere, it is within each one of us.—BLACK ELK

ONENESS

In Black Elk's great vision, we are all connected to each other by the common center we all share. You carry the Great Spirit inside you, at the center of yourself, and it is always there, even when you're not paying attention to it. Knowing that you carry the Spirit inside you makes you at peace. Going further with this powerful idea, you could say that you declare war on yourself when you start pretending you are not one with anything. If you say you are not one with anger or fear or sexuality or any aspect of yourself or the world, a rattle of disharmony begins that soon sends an unpleasant vibration through the whole neighborhood of the billions of cells whose dance you are. Peace only comes when you declare yourself one again with all.

■ A CONSCIOUS LIVING PRACTICE FOR TODAY ■

Take a moment right now to feel your connection with everything. Feel how your body, though made up of many separate parts, is actually all one. Feel how you are exactly the same as all other human beings— all humanity is one. Feel how there is no "you" separate from the universe itself. It's all one thing, and you are it. As you move through your life today, focus on the oneness rather than the separateness of things.

If your basic contact with essence is dammed up, your creativity often goes underground or is misdirected, even squandered . . .

UNCOVERING YOURSELF

You are focusing on uncovering yourself to yourself, on looking in the mirror and the soul and allowing yourself to know acceptance for what you see. Many of you spend your life in the struggle to hold down the secret shame that runs in the river of your blood, coloring everything in dark, hidden tones. Now you have chosen to tell the microscopic truth; you have chosen full expression and holding nothing back. Your starting point is with yourself and you will be your first audience. I do not promise that telling the truth causes no fallout, within yourself or in relationship with others. I *do* promise the fresh, exhilarating breath of joy and the life-affirming power of making a free choice.

■ A CONSCIOUS LIVING PRACTICE FOR TODAY ■

Let yourself know something that makes you feel discomfort. Sit with the knowledge and let it take you in. Embrace it and the feelings that result and ask yourself, "How do I feel, loving that which I believed to be unlovable?"

The quickest way to make yourself miserable is to stop keeping your agreements. Then you have to pretend you don't notice, or you have to tell lies and make excuses to cover yourself. Next thing you know, you're in the ditch and not sure how you got there.

—GAIL PADILLA

THE FINE ART OF AGREEMENTS

One of the skills of conscious living is making and keeping your agreements. Not keeping agreements you make—and making agreements you don't intend to keep—drains energy and detracts from the forward progress of your life. You end up spending so much time handling broken agreements that you don't have creative energy left for successful living. The clear analogy, and one most of you recognize, is with a lie. Think about the energy required to develop and maintain the subterfuge necessary to support a lie. First, the lie itself: Is it believable? Is your body telling the same story that is coming from your lips? And then the world: Are you managing the world in such a way as to be certain that your lie is not exposed? Lying is hard work, and worse, unproductive.

The bare essentials: Think carefully before you make an agreement. Make only agreements you really want to make. Scrupulously keep the ones you make. If you need to change one, do it promptly and consciously, and be willing to listen to others' feelings about your change to the agreement.

■ A CONSCIOUS LIVING PRACTICE FOR TODAY ■

Make a list of the agreements you've broken or changed over the past week. Go to each person and say, "I want to acknowledge that I broke an agreement with you. I'd like to know if you need or want anything from me about that."

If making a list seems daunting, just think of one agreement you've broken and make amends with that one person. I predict that you will be amazed at the amount of creative energy you'll recover from the interaction.

....

Our life is frittered away by detail . . . simplify, simplify.—HENRY DAVID THOREAU

STREAMLINING AND SIMPLIFYING

One of the most powerful things you can do during your year of conscious living is to examine all aspects of your life in light of the question "Am I operating at the level of simplicity I want?" You don't have to be austere or sell all your belongings—the only measure is whether your level of simplicity is satisfying to you. A few years back I realized that the complexity of my life was consuming too much energy. My wife and I had accumulated three cars, two houses, an office building, and a host of other "necessities." It seemed that a remarkable amount of time and energy was spent handling repairs, scheduling helpers, dealing with staff problems, and so forth. Finally we saw the folly of our ways and began a process of simplifying. Now we have streamlined to one car and one house and one office. We have become much happier and more productive by living in the question "Will this course of action simplify or complicate my life?"

■ A CONSCIOUS LIVING PRACTICE FOR TODAY ■

Study your closet for a few moments today. Quickly note the clothes you absolutely love to wear. Notice which ones you simply put up with. Consider the bold step of getting rid of all the clothes you don't love to wear. Invite some friends over for a "shopping" spree. Then notice what happens to your mood and energy level after you shift to wearing only clothes you love.

The greatest griefs are those we call ourselves.—SOPHOCLES

POWERFUL LESSONS

If we're paying attention, we can learn the most powerful lessons easily and comfortably. If we're not paying attention, we seem to require the same lessons to be administered "the hard way."

Here's an example: I once had the opportunity to hear a speech by a personnel executive who had hired and fired thousands of people in his life. He said something that made my ears stand to attention: It was his experience that being fired was one of the best things that could happen to a person. He had followed the careers of thousands of people who had been fired, and he had never seen anybody who'd been harmed by it. Thinking I'd misheard him, I sought him out afterward to answer some of my questions. He elaborated that when people get fired, they're forced to wake up. He had been surprised to find that people tend to get the message. Following the firing, they change careers or go back to school, or pursue the dream they've been putting off, or embark on any number of new paths. Probably, he said, being fired gives people impetus to do what they've wanted to do all along.

My own experience fits his exactly. I've been fired from one job in my career. I hated the place I was working and the petty tyrant who ran the agency. Being fired inspired me to go back to graduate school to get my Ph.D., a move I'd been putting off because I thought I couldn't afford it. I made the decision to go, and right away I found the money to do it.

■ A CONSCIOUS LIVING PRACTICE FOR TODAY ■

Ask yourself a few key questions: Are there dreams you're putting off? Decisions you need to make? Paths you ought to be following? Are you waiting for life to teach you "the hard way," or are you open to learning easefully?

FEBRUARY

Life can only take place in the present moment.—BUDDHA

A SIMPLE FORMULA FOR CONSCIOUS LIVING

A graduate student in a class I was teaching a few years ago asked me a great question: If you could put a slogan on a T-shirt that everyone wore, what would the slogan say? In essence, she was asking for the simplest possible summation of the principles of conscious living. I came up with two, then the class joined in and we had a stimulating brainstorming session in which they came up with variations of their own. My first one was: Feel all your feelings, tell all your truth, and keep all your agreements. My second one was: Feel what you feel, get clear on your purpose, and do what needs to be done.

It's important in life to feel all your feelings, but don't stop there. You may wake up the morning you're to give a big speech with a sore throat and a deep conviction that you don't want to do it. Purely listening to your feelings might keep you in bed. But you also need to be clear on your purpose. Perhaps your purpose, when you really tune in to it, is to provide leadership to the organization you're speaking to. Even in light of your feelings, your purpose will get you out of bed and out the door to do what needs to be done.

■ A CONSCIOUS LIVING PRACTICE FOR TODAY ■

Think ahead to the next few days. Is there anything you have resistance to doing? If so, focus on it for a moment. Feel all your feelings about it, then get clear on your purpose for doing it. If your purpose feels sound, commit yourself to doing it and feeling all your feelings about it.

FEBRUARY 2

I like dreams of the future better than the history of the past.—THOMAS JEFFERSON

TAPPING ENERGY

Some people are pushed from behind by the past, while others are drawn forward by the pull of the future. Which is more powerful? Which is more pleasurable?

One way to answer this question is to think of a farm image. Have you ever seen a horse pushing a wagon? Probably not. Take a moment, though, to imagine it. Not only doesn't the image make sense at an intellectual level, but it probably strikes you as absurd at a gut level (a level you should pay attention to and listen to more intuitively, as animals listen for the change in the tone of the wind and feel the electric charge in the air as a tornado approaches).

There is a great deal more power in the pull of the future—if you can let go of the past long enough to tap it.

■ A CONSCIOUS LIVING PRACTICE FOR TODAY ■

Let's reach far into the future to harness its power: Imagine being on your deathbed, still lucid and in a philosophical mood, when a visitor drops in to see you. Your visitor asks you, "Was your life a complete success?" Without hesitation, you answer yes! Your visitor asks, "What did you experience or accomplish that made your life a total success?" Again, without hesitation, you name off four or five things you did or experienced that made your life a journey of complete fulfillment. What are they?

FEBRUARY 3

Such as we are made of, such we be.——WILLIAM SHAKESPEARE

OF WHAT ARE YOU MADE?

Of what are you made? Are you made of the memories of your past and the realities of your present and the wishes for your future? What have you been and what will you be? The miracle is that *the answer is yours to create.* You will be that which you decide to be. Make up your mind to tell the microscopic truth and you will be honest. Vow to enjoy full closeness in your life and to clear up anything that stands in the way of that closeness, and it will be yours. Commit to your own complete development as an individual and you will see your commitment bear fruit. The magic of conscious living is that it is within your power to create it; with commitment and the proper tools, you are on your way to the conscious life.

■ A CONSCIOUS LIVING PRACTICE FOR TODAY ■

It is up to you to decide the path you will take in your life. One of the first steps is to ask yourself the right questions in order to see your path more clearly.

Spend a few moments today thinking about one word that best describes what you most want in the following relationship areas.

- Family
- Work
- Friendship
- Partner

At every single moment of one's life, one is going to be no less than what one has been.
—OSCAR WILDE

WHAT MAKES YOU REAL

Laura writes, from a foreign hotel room: Ada, the housekeeper, is cleaning around me. We make an attempt at communication but soon fall silent; we speak different languages. Ada picks up a framed picture of my children that sits by the bed, and we both smile and settle for exchanging names and the number of children we have, since *niño* is the only Spanish word I know, and she seems to know no English. When she leaves I realize that I am both cheered and frustrated by our attempts at communication. I am cheered because I was feeling lonely and connection-starved, and even our pointing and gesturing and smiles were a connection, but I am also frustrated because I couldn't say or understand more. So much about conscious loving is about developing a shared language, a way to know and be known. When you are in a foreign land—literally or figuratively—where you are not known, you are reminded that human communication is what makes you real.

■ A CONSCIOUS LIVING PRACTICE FOR TODAY ■

Think about a person who has brought joy to you simply by existing. Whether in person or in writing, tell this person of his or her importance to you, being particularly conscious of not focusing on what she or he does for you but instead on what she or he *is* to you.

You need to recognize that the best thing to do with feelings is to feel them.

FEBRUARY 5

The deepest principle in human nature is the craving to be appreciated.

—WILLIAM JAMES

THE ART OF APPRECIATION

One recurring theme you will discover in your year of living consciously is the art of appreciation. I cannot stress the value of appreciation enough. All it takes is one second of pure appreciation, followed by a clear expression of it, to send a relationship on a soaring spiral of positivity. It has become unpopular to do so in our cynical world; people roll their eyes and mutter "Pollyanna" at someone who regularly manages to find appreciation and positivity in the world. Many of you are hedging your bets, waiting for something good to happen *before* you express appreciation. This is the wrong way to go about it. Go out looking for things to appreciate—starting with the way things are, whether that reality is convenient for you or not—and riches will begin to flow toward you in ever-widening circles.

■ A CONSCIOUS LIVING PRACTICE FOR TODAY ■

Take three deep breaths—slow, full, easy breaths. Feel appreciation for yourself for ten seconds. Give yourself deep, rich appreciation for no good reason. Just appreciate yourself for the sheer pleasure of it. Now, think of one thing you really appreciate about someone you know. Find a way to get the appreciation to them within the next hour: a letter, a call, an e-mail. Watch what happens to the relationship—I predict that you will be pleasantly surprised.

FEBRUARY 6

All the knowledge I possess everyone else can acquire, but my heart is all my own.
—GOETHE

DEFINING YOURSELF

What you have experienced and done, your history, often defines who you are. I have already discussed letting go of the judgment and blame you might assign based on your past while recognizing that you can't actually rid yourself of your personal history. If you are to have relationship knowledge, you must listen to the outward voices and to your intuition, your inward voice. You know what you think and feel, and you know what you see and experience; merging these things and learning to treat them as the truth is another step on your path to knowledge and essence.

A starting point on this journey of defining yourself begins with the act of putting down the pen with which you rewrite your story. That failed marriage that wasn't your fault? The drinking problem that you were driven to by circumstances beyond your control? Your tendency to have bosses who are easily irritated, thus keeping you from career advancement? Imagine, for a moment, the blissful freedom of coming at these things from the other side, the side in which you claim yourself (warts and all) and make peace with yourself and your personal history.

■ A CONSCIOUS LIVING PRACTICE FOR TODAY ■

When you are centered, your breath will tell you so. Take as long as you need to slow down, close your eyes, and breathe deeply, until you can feel a place in the very core of your abdomen begin to absorb the peace and good feeling that clean breathing brings. Stay there comfortably for a while once you arrive, allowing yourself to know that sense of well-being.

Each moment requires you to choose commitment or complacency.

Things like being right and faultfinding have a seductive quality to them; people frequently use them like a drug.

THE TIES THAT BIND

Who among you doesn't claim a habit you would wish to break? Have you ever heard people talk about their habits? The half-proud, half-rueful words make their habits sound like lovably, if unruly, pets. "I know I shouldn't," says one person, while another nods and says, "I'm going to stop on New Year's." Who's being fooled here?

Killing habits aside—smoking, drinking too much, using drugs, beating down your feelings until they cower inside, afraid to be heard—not one among us doesn't have the ghosts of habit whirling around inside, ephemeral and unfriendly. *Know your ghosts, and you will know that the enemy is often within.*

■ A CONSCIOUS LIVING PRACTICE FOR TODAY ■

Identify a relationship habit that you have that others have often commented upon. Spend a moment thinking about where that habit originated, and then think carefully about the purposes it might serve in your relationships. If you find yourself thinking that it serves no purpose, think again. Everything you do, you do for a reason. This is perhaps most true when your actions seem to betray you again and again.

FEBRUARY 8

Habits are first cobwebs, then cables.—SPANISH PROVERB

GIVING VOICE TO YOUR LIFE

Since the advent of psychoanalysis, also known as "talk therapy," implicit in its approach has been the concept of remembering and giving voice to experiences in order to understand present relationships and the behaviors and neuroses that occur within those relationships. I believe in the importance of memory, particularly in the lasting impressions made by birth experiences, but too often I have seen therapy stop once a connection is made between the past and the present, as if to remember is to change. This is not so. That your heart knows everything it has experienced from birth on is true, but the idea that culling that knowledge from the dusty corners of your heart will create strong, loving, conscious relationships doesn't necessarily follow. You must do something with the secrets and truths you bring forth, translating them into present-day realities.

■ A CONSCIOUS LIVING PRACTICE FOR TODAY ■

Think about this sentence for a moment: I have heard from family or family friends who knew me when I was very young that my dominant personality traits were _____ .

How have you continued to see yourself as you were defined early on? How have these prophecies of others continued to define you?

It is no use walking anywhere to preach unless our walking is our preaching.
—St. Francis of Assisi

ENJOYING THE PROCESS

One of the most important learnings in your year of living consciously will likely be this: The joy of the journey itself is not only a key goal, it is *the* goal. The outcomes of the journey, whatever they are, will always be in the zone of the unknown. While you're getting to where you're going, though, you will have the opportunity to enjoy the greatest show on earth, the moment-by-moment process of consciousness itself. I once asked a revered Tibetan lama to define his most important teaching. Without hesitation he said, "Richness. Richness means that every moment you are blessed with a free abundance of thoughts—the flow of consciousness itself. Who could ask for more?" I replied, "What you call 'richness' is the same thing that a lot of people think is driving them nuts." The lama nodded, a sly smile forming on his lips, and said, "I know. Better to call it 'richness,' don't you think?"

■ A CONSCIOUS LIVING PRACTICE FOR TODAY ■

As you go through your day, observe richness flowing through your mind, the free and abundant stream of thoughts. Observe richness in your body, the flow of sensation and feeling. Enjoy your riches as you use your mind and body all day long.

FEBRUARY 10

Believe nothing, no matter where you read it or who said it—even if I have said it—
unless it agrees with your own reason and your own common sense.—BUDDHA

THE UNCOMMON ART OF COMMON SENSE

Many of the great teachers of conscious living over the past two thousand years have had trouble with the orthodoxy. Socrates met his fate for "corrupting the youth of Athens" with his ideas, and Epictetus had to leave his school behind when a wave of early Christian fundamentalism swept through Rome. But you don't have to look back into history—or even outside of yourself—for the battle between the orthodox (from a word that means "straight-thinking") and the heretical (from a word that means "to think for yourself"). Most of you have an orthodox and a heretic living right inside your own mind. On a daily basis I spot the thinking of my inner orthodox, who wants to follow the rules, to be right and do things the tried-and-true way. Even though I value thinking for myself above almost anything else, I find I must work hard to keep my inner heretic alive and well. Is the same true for you?

■ A CONSCIOUS LIVING PRACTICE FOR TODAY ■

Take a few breaths and get centered. Acknowledge your inner orthodox and your inner heretic: Say to yourself, "I like to be right and I like to be free." Make friends with both sides of yourself.

....

FEBRUARY 11

The great danger for most of us is not that our aim is too high and we miss it,
but that it is too low and we reach it.—MICHELANGELO

THINKING BIG

I once sat in a coffee shop with a friend, counseling (and consoling) him. The friend was a million dollars in debt, he said, and he couldn't see any way out besides more hard work. But that was the same way of thinking that had gotten him where he was, and he was suspicious of doing more of the same. Did I have any suggestions? I asked him: What would be the biggest, most inspiring goal you could imagine? To invent something that would benefit humanity, he replied, his face lighting up in a big smile. Using table napkins, we generated a list of possible inventions in his area of expertise. Ten years after this conversation, his net worth is approaching fifty million dollars from just one of the ideas on that napkin, and he's working on a couple of others.

■ A CONSCIOUS LIVING PRACTICE FOR TODAY ■

Ask yourself: What grand goals would inspire me every minute of every day? What would I do with my life if I were playing full-out? If I were thinking big—AND EVEN BIGGER THAN THAT!—what dream would I commit to fulfilling?

....

FEBRUARY 12
A stumble may prevent a fall.—ENGLISH PROVERB

YOUR JOURNEY OF CHANGE

Are you expecting to make your journey of change without mistakes? If you are, I rejoice, because you have already made your first mistake—in thinking that the path to a conscious heart and to conscious relationship is one without pitfalls. I rejoice because, of course, to err is human, and I am most comfortable with others when they are most human. But I also celebrate your mistake because it speaks of optimism, of a hopefulness that will carry you through the mistakes and obstacles bound to occur along your path.

On February 8, you focused on some of the ways in which people described you as a child, and how those descriptions continue to influence your self-view even now.

Today, think about the first instances in which you recall being censored or censured for those same qualities by which others defined you so frequently.

....

FEBRUARY 13

Trust me, but look to thyself.——IRISH PROVERB

THE FALLACY OF SAFETY

Those "safe," protected places you create around your heart—the ones designed so that no one can hurt you—have one fatal flaw: if they protect you, they can also wall you off. I am careful to put quotation marks around the word *safe* because I have learned the fallacy in that word. In the real world of conscious relationship, no one and everyone is safe. What does this mean? It is a paradox, because in a truly connected, committed, and honest relationship, you put your heart out there right in the thick of things, and the possibility certainly exists that your heart may end up bruised and battered. On the other hand, if you don't put your heart out in your relationships, I can guarantee that it will not only bruise, like fruit that is over-ripe but not partaken of, it will wither and grow bitter. So, while you may—and, in fact, you are likely to—experience pain as the result of your new connectedness, you will also have the opportunity, time and again, to experience soaring joy and a degree of good feeling that may well seem unimaginable to the person with the hiding heart.

Continuing with the work of the past several days, focus once again on your early character traits and your first memories of being censored for those traits. Today, pick the one that first came to your mind and think of the ways in which this trait manifests itself in you now, in your adult life and relationships.

If you find yourself thinking that this trait does not manifest itself in you now, I suggest that you may have merely cloaked it in another name.

....

FEBRUARY 14

If there is anything we wish to change in the child, we should first examine it and see whether it is not something that could better be changed in ourselves.—CARL G. JUNG

MONSTERS BENEATH THE BED

Laura remember months of dealing on a nightly basis with monsters under the bed of her three-year-old. She writes: I should have known that there really *were* monsters because my son told me it was true with those earnest, frightened eyes. Still, I have to admit, I wasn't a believer (I was, after all, an *adult*, and don't adults know that there are no monsters?). "Don't cry," I would plead. "There aren't any monsters. There is no such thing as a monster." I don't know where my training in empathic listening went during those late-night monster episodes; perhaps it was hiding, impossibly, under the bed with those hulking, scary creatures. In any case, after weeks and weeks of this, one night I took his hands and looked into his eyes and said, "Monsters are very scary, aren't they?" He nodded solemnly and we searched the bedroom together, proving that they weren't there. "They must have gone home to sleep in their monster beds," I observed. "I bet their monster mommies tucked them in." Another solemn—and sleepy—nod. Soon he was asleep, breathing deeply and peacefully. All Benjamin wanted was to be heard and to be believed, to know that I understood and honored his fear. He didn't have the words to be able to say that the dark, the perceived abandonment of nighttime, frightened his little soul, and so the monsters came instead to serve as his voice. For so many of you, your earliest experiences, time and again, were like the one in my son's room when the monsters still visited. "Don't cry," your parents said, and their words implied, "You don't know what you're feeling." Your work now is twofold: first, you must make the journey back to believing that you *do* know what you're feeling; second, you must make the commitment to honoring the feelings of others with whom you have a relationship, without imposing upon them your own version of reality.

■ A CONSCIOUS LIVING PRACTICE FOR TODAY ■

Continuing on with your recent work, identify several ways in which you have taken on the censoring/censuring role with yourself. Notice how you respond when you exhibit the traits that garnered you disapproval early on in life.

FEBRUARY 15

Love is a fruit in season at all times, and within the reach of every hand.
—MOTHER TERESA OF CALCUTTA

MOMENTS OF POTENTIAL

You become who you are by the ways you handle moments of potential intimacy. The course of your life is shaped by those moments in which you either open yourself to intimacy or shrink away from it in fear or despair as some voice from the past warns you off, as if to be happy is to be safe. There's that word again: *safe!* You create your destiny by dealing with the grip of longing. And yet, for so many of you, the voices layered on your longing are voices of warning, telling you that longing is a dangerous business, one that will get you into all sorts of trouble if you let it guide you. Unfortunately, many of you unconsciously listen to that voice and thus sentence yourself to a destiny of loneliness and lack of fulfillment. By not knowing which way to turn at the crucial crossroads of destiny that confront you hourly, you lose your way and often do not get back home again.

■ A CONSCIOUS LIVING PRACTICE FOR TODAY ■

Think about a crucial crossroads of decision in your life. Of the choices you made as to which path to take, think now about the two that seemed most obvious and likely at the time. Often, the first choice that occurs to you comes from the heart. The second choice is often heavy with the voice of reason, your conscience, your programming.

Which did you choose to follow?

Looking back now, what might have happened if you had chosen to follow the other voice—whichever one you didn't choose?

....

FEBRUARY 16

We were deliberately designed to learn by trial and error.
We're brought up, unfortunately, to think that nobody should make mistakes. Most children are degeniused by the love and fear of their parents—that they might make a mistake.
—BUCKMINSTER FULLER

THE POWER OF BEING WRONG MOST OF THE TIME

Buckminster Fuller was onced asked how he continued to be so creative throughout his life, registering patents for inventions up into his eighties. Without hesitation he replied that it was because he was willing to make more mistakes than anyone he'd ever met! The automatic pilot of an airplane is a remarkable device for at least two reasons: First, it gets you to your destination by being wrong most of the time. Second, it does so because it self-corrects thousands of times without losing its temper. It just notices it's wrong, corrects itself, then does the whole process over again a second or two later.

■ A CONSCIOUS LIVING PRACTICE FOR TODAY ■

Today, go out in search of mistakes. Rather than resist making mistakes, get willing to make as many as you make *and* learn from them cheerfully. Life is not about not making mistakes—it's about learning and making more so you can learn even more.

....

FEBRUARY 17

The stream of creation and dissolution never stops.—HERACLITUS

HOLDING YOUR FEELINGS LIGHTLY

One of my friends has a saying that he claims is the secret to happiness: Don't squeeze your feelings. He means that when you're feeling happy, don't try to hold on to it, and when you're feeling down, don't try to keep from feeling it. Give all your feelings—both the ups and downs—room to breathe, and, like breath, they will pass quickly.

I was stuck in a traffic jam a while back, feeling hot and irritable because I was late for a meeting. Suddenly I remembered, "Don't squeeze your feelings." I took a breath and let myself feel irritated. A few seconds later my feelings shifted toward the pleasant, and, as if by magic, the traffic moved.

The moment you start taking your feelings too seriously, you get a grip on them and they get a grip on you. When you lighten up your grip on them, they get room to breathe, and so do you.

Make a commitment to holding your feelings lightly as you move through your day. Initiate a thought such as, "I commit to giving all my feelings room to breathe today. I allow myself to feel all my feelings when I feel them, and I allow them to pass through without interference."

....

FEBRUARY 18

The great man is he who does not lose his child-heart.—MENCIUS

SEEING THROUGH TO THE CHILD

In one of Graham Greene's novels, an elderly priest describes what he has learned from a lifetime of hearing confessions. One lesson is: There's no such thing as a grown-up. This perception can be helpful when dealing with conflict situations. I once hepled three powerful executives iron out a corporate snag they'd hit that was costing them millions of dollars a week. We had been going back and forth for several hours, with no real resolution of the issues, when suddenly I had a vision that brought an inner smile to me. I shifted from seeing them as middle-aged men in hand-tailored suits to seeing them as little boys in a schoolyard. This shift in perception allowed me an insight: One of them was a bully and the other two were scared of him but smarter than he was. As soon as I realized this, I could speak to the fears running as undercurrents in the situation. Resolution was reached within an hour.

■ A CONSCIOUS LIVING PRACTICE FOR TODAY ■

Take a few minutes to think of several key people in your life. As you reflect on each of them, ask yourself what they may have been like as children. Imagine their childhood faces, and tune in to their childhood fears and dreams.

Now, do the same for yourself.

Taking a conscious stand for enjoyment is very important, because many of us have strong beliefs that relationships have to be effortful, painful, and difficult.

YOUR LONGING TO CONNECT

You are not alone in your longing to connect, to love, to be loved for who you truly are. Who knows, though, who you truly are? Do you hide it from others because the darkness in your soul is too shameful to be seen? And do you hide your longing, too, when it grips you? Do you reach for something, anything (the remote control, a box of candy, a beer, a cigarette) when your heart constricts with longing? The way you relax that constriction, the fist in your chest, will tell you and the world all you need to know about who you are when it comes to longing. If you relax the fist and make connections with others, you will become happy, free, productive. If you don't, no honors or accolades, no material goods that you acquire like blankets to warm your cold heart, will ever fill the void created by longing. Only one thing fills that void, and that is true, honest connection with other human beings.

■ A CONSCIOUS LIVING PRACTICE FOR TODAY ■

Close your eyes and spend a moment focusing on your breath and on the sensations in your chest. Feel your rib cage where it rounds your sides. Is it tight? Is it wrapped around your tender organs—and especially your heart—like a protective fence? Does it move easily and comfortably as you inhale and exhale, or does it seem to resist your breath? Now, focus on your heart; let yourself become aware of its presence in your chest. Breathing deeply, simply know your heart—its rhythms, its patterns, its color, its strength.

Infinite riches in a little room . . . ——CHRISTOPHER MARLOWE

HAVE AN "OUT OF YOURSELF" EXPERIENCE

Many people get trapped inside their own personas, especially as they approach midlife. They find themselves unwilling to do things outside their own worldview. Gradually their circle of friends gets tighter, the range of experiences they enjoy more limited. Unless they do something to shake themselves up (benignly, if possible), the circle can become a noose.

An antidote to rigidity is to do things outside of your experience, things you wouldn't ordinarily do. For example, I learn a new musical instrument every year or two. My wife, once afraid of flying, overcame her fear by going parachuting. Two elders of my acquaintance set the goal of going to at least one foreign country each year in their seventies and eighties, and they're sticking to their plan so far. Their philosophy of aging is "Use it or lose it." They go out of their way to keep the circle expanding rather than shrinking.

■ A CONSCIOUS LIVING PRACTICE FOR TODAY ■

Take some time today to think of several things that would be "totally unlike you" but that you secretly suspect would be very good for you. Generate a list of these, post them publicly, then *do them!*

To me, every hour of the light and dark is a miracle.—WALT WHITMAN

PROBABILITY AND LIKELIHOOD

The beauty of following a path of conscious living is the joy of making miracles a part of your everyday reality. You come to see them for what they are, probability and likelihood in your hands. We sometimes think of miracles as rare birds, things bestowed on us from above, but let's break out of that limited perspective. Think of miracles as everyday acts you can perform.

Because of my work, I get to see the miracle of change up close every day. Yesterday I watched smiles break out on the faces of a couple who had come in an hour before with the sour grimaces of long-term relationship conflict. She told him the truth about some of her hurts and angers. He, with some coaching, listened to her in a new way—without judging her. Something as simple as a new way of listening to each other sent them out hand in hand. Seeing those smiles break out was as much of a miracle to me as the first blossom of springtime must be to a gardener.

■ A CONSCIOUS LIVING PRACTICE FOR TODAY ■

Promise yourself a miracle today. When you become aware that you're judging or censoring yourself today, suspend that thought. Take a few deep breaths instead. Inhale slowly . . . exhale slowly. Then look around you with fresh eyes . . . listen with new ears. You may find that you are standing in a field of miracles right where you are.

Everything in nature contains all the power of nature.
Everything is made of one hidden stuff.—RALPH WALDO EMERSON

YOUR UNIVERSAL CONNECTION

One of the most powerful and practical concepts of conscious living is that you are connected to everything else in the universe. If you assume that we are all made of the same stuff—whatever it is—this means that there is one unbroken chain of creation of which we are an equal part. It means that we are all made of the infinite intelligence that pervades everything. The practical use of this idea is that you can work out all the truly important issues in your life by opening up to this inner intelligence. No one can know the power of this gift until they have opened to trusting it completely.

I did a session a while back with a woman who had a terrible headache when she came in. She'd carried it for several days, and even a visit to her doctor for stronger medicine hadn't helped much. I invited her to give it a different medicine, ten seconds of nonjudgmental attention. Simply "feel the sensations without judging them," was the way I put it. That ten seconds led her to a realization: She had been angry for days at her partner for refusing to do a small favor my client had asked. I then invited her to give her anger ten seconds of nonjudgmental attention. As she did this her eyes opened wide. "It's disappearing," she said, with genuine wonder in her voice. Within the next twenty minutes the headache subsided to the size of a walnut, then a pinhead, then nothing. All from ten seconds of nonjudgmental attention.

■ A CONSCIOUS LIVING PRACTICE FOR TODAY ■

Purely as an experiment, recruit the infinite intelligence of the universe to assist you in solving a specific problem. Select some problem, concern, or issue that you've been unable to resolve as yet through your usual means. Keeping the problem in mind, invite a solution by initiating a thought such as, "I surrender this problem to be resolved through my connection to infinite intelligence. I invoke its power in opening me to an innovative solution." Then forget about it and go on about your business. Notice what happens over the next few days.

....

FEBRUARY 23

The curious paradox is that when I accept myself just as I am, then I can change.
—CARL ROGERS

THE MAGICAL ROOT CANAL

While in the thick of finishing a project, Laura was ignoring severe pain in a tooth. She writes: I've had lots of serious dental work (twelve root canals to date) because of a car accident ten years ago. Although I've had some great dentists, I dread going for dental work because it's painful and it seems to always require extensive work (and money). I rarely need a simple filling. When I couldn't ignore this tooth anymore, I went to a new dentist, and, not surprisingly, I needed a root canal. When the dentist began the procedure, I let myself sink down into relaxation, breathing and not resisting the pain. This wasn't something I'd tried before; I'd always tensed up and experienced root canals as awful, sometimes excruciating. Each time I began to feel pain this time, I relaxed, allowing the pain to wash over me instead of resisting it. After about ten minutes, I no longer tensed up; I was in a different zone and the pain ceased entirely. The dentist was having a tough time finding the infected nerve, but I was so relaxed that at some point I knew, intuitively, that he was at the nerve, although I felt no pain. I urged him to continue; if he returned to where he'd been, I said, he'd find the nerve. He watched me carefully and when I again had the sensation—not pain, just knowing—I raised my eyebrows. A short pull and, sure enough, he had the nerve.

He was amazed. He'd never had the experience of a patient being able to tell him by intuition when the nerve was contacted—except through pain. Neither had I. He had trusted me enough, though, to take what I said and act on it. I can't say I'm looking forward to the next root canal (I'm conscious, but not crazy!), but I'm not *afraid* of it, either. I know what to do now. Stop resisting the pain. Flow with it instead of fighting or fleeing from it. Just breathe. Just flow.

■ A CONSCIOUS LIVING PRACTICE FOR TODAY ■

The next time you hurt yourself, notice how you respond. You probably tense up and have a surge of adrenalin. Try the following things and notice how differently you experience the pain:

- Breathe slowly and deeply, focusing your thoughts on counting each breath.
- Relax your muscles entirely, letting your arms hang limp by your side.
- Visualize the pain as waves washing over you, neither good nor bad, simply there, something that you cannot fight, something that will recede.

....

FEBRUARY 24

The great charm in argument is really finding one's own opinions, not other people's.
—EVELYN WAUGH

RELATIONSHIP CONFLICTS

Let's take apart the essence of a miracle in relationship. First, I will examine a typical pattern in a relationship conflict, one that is likely to be familiar to you. You come home from work tired and stressed, and your partner arrives at the same time and asks what's for dinner. It doesn't matter which gender I assign to each partner; either could ask the question. You feel a tightness form in your belly and that fist makes itself known in your chest. You answer your partner sarcastically, perhaps saying, "I don't know; maybe you should check with our cook." Your partner responds with equal sarcasm; it's not important what he or she says, just that it stings. And off you go, on your way down the path of that conflict that you can't believe two intelligent, caring adults have been having for countless years now.

■ A CONSCIOUS LIVING PRACTICE FOR TODAY ■

Answer the following questions in your mind:

- An argument that I frequently have with my partner is about
  _____.

- When the argument is beginning my belly feels _____.
- When the argument is beginning my chest feels _____.
- I know the argument is in full swing once I hear myself say
  _____.

- I know the argument is in full swing once I hear my partner say
  _____.

What might you learn by your answers?

....

FEBRUARY 25

It is possible to feel the flow of loving feeling—inside your body and between you and others—nearly all the time.

OFF AND RUNNING

Let's look at the inner workings of that same argument about dinner. You walked into the situation with some strong physical sensations at work: tension, tiredness, stress. Perhaps your partner was experiencing similar sensations; let's assume so here. Your partner asked a question about dinner, which triggered physical sensations in your body: a tightness in your belly and tension, in the form of a fist, in your chest, and a defensive stance from you. Ignoring those feelings, you replied sarcastically and your partner defensively responded in kind. Within about ten seconds, the argument was off and running as you wondered why the two of you couldn't get past what seems, on the surface, like a somewhat inconsequential issue.

■ A CONSCIOUS LIVING PRACTICE FOR TODAY ■

Review for a moment some of the communication patterns and behaviors that could notify you that you are in a ten-second window of opportunity in a conflict with your partner.

Make a commitment to yourself: *I will be aware of the many chances to change that which does not work in my relationships. Whatever I withdraw from, or whatever I go toward and embrace, becomes the universe that I have created.*

....

FEBRUARY 26
Too often we enjoy the comfort of opinion without the discomfort of thought.
—JOHN F. KENNEDY

CREATING A FAVORABLE CLIMATE

Using the same situation that you have been considering for several days now, let's identify how to create a favorable climate for a miracle. Think of your conflict as a greenhouse. If you keep the climate temperate for the roots of your relationship, you will encourage growth and flowering; if you ignore the need to do so and attempt to keep it comfortable, in the method of old patterns, for only yourself, a withering will take place. In this example, had you allowed yourself to be notified by your physical sensations (tightness in the belly, a fist in the chest) and your emotional experience (defensiveness), you would have alerted yourself that you were in a ten-second window. Instead of getting defensive, you would have wondered. Wondering opens the door to the zone of the miraculous, taking you out of the zone of the known and into the field of possibility, where miracles can occur. "I feel as if you assume that dinner is my responsibility," you might say, "and I wonder why that makes me feel so angry and defensive. I have a sick feeling in my stomach at even hearing your dinner question." There is nothing you have said, then, that your partner can take apart or argue with; each statement contained an unarguable truth.

■ A CONSCIOUS LIVING PRACTICE FOR TODAY ■

Think again on a frequent conflict with your partner, and allow yourself to wonder rather than worry. Here's how it works.

If you are worrying, you are feeling fear, perhaps about what might happen if you share your feelings truthfully (might you be abandoned, disliked, unloved, criticized?).

If you are wondering, you are asking yourself this simple question: I wonder what this conflict is about for me, since I need to be in it again and again?

....

FEBRUARY 27
You can't step into the same river twice.——HERACLITUS

WINDOWS OF OPPORTUNITY

Continuing yesterday's example: By wondering, you made a crucial choice during the window of opportunity, the ten-second window. You didn't get defensive. You didn't allow yourself to be carried along by your assumptions and past experiences without checking in with your partner. Instead, you wondered. Wondering opens the door to the zone of the miraculous. Next, you opened up to your feelings, noting to your partner that you felt angry and defensive. By working through this process, you will not only attempt miracles, you will make them happen. By focusing on unarguable truths and by giving them a voice, you will be one breath away from creating a miracle in the most significant area of your life, your relationship to others.

■ A CONSCIOUS LIVING PRACTICE FOR TODAY ■

Identify several unarguable truths about yourself. It doesn't matter what area of your life they are about, only that they are true.

Spend a few moments, right now, simply sitting with these truths. Breathe slowly and deeply as you acknowledge the truths, and feel how it is to know these things about yourself. Do not judge, do not intellectualize, do not do anything but feel the truth about yourself.

The only way to deepen and go forward in a close relationship is through becoming more transparent.

....

FEBRUARY 28

Shall I, like a hermit, dwell on a rock or in a cell?—SIR WALTER RALEIGH

RECOGNIZING OPPORTUNITIES FOR CHANGE

How do you recognize an opportunity (what I call a ten-second window) for relationship change when it comes along? The good news is that there are a number of different ways to recognize these ten-second windows of opportunity, so if you miss one cue, you're likely to see another (and besides, you've just committed to not being perfect anymore, so you'll be welcoming mistakes anyway, reframing them into learning windows). A clear cue that I have seen countless times—one you've seen too—is in what is called "affect." You see an expression on someone's face that alerts you to the possibility for change. You see that it is *your* responsibility to do the noticing; the window is less about the expression and more about your relationship alertness. You've probably used this window many times already; you're giving someone directions, say, and you observe a confused look: eyes squinty, mouth puckering, head shaking slightly. You say, "I notice you shaking your head. What's up?" In a more emotional example you might gentle your words, saying something like, "I notice something in your expression. I'm wondering what you're feeling right now."

■ A CONSCIOUS LIVING PRACTICE FOR TODAY ■

In your next three interactions with your partner or another significant other, open yourself to the window of affect. Watch your partner's expression closely as you talk—regardless of the topic—and if you see his or her expression change, try noticing it and wondering about it to yourself. Simply try out the language within your head, getting familiar with it. Remind yourself that you do not make guesses as to the feelings being experienced (i.e., "I notice that you look sad") nor are there any judgments ("I'm wondering if you're angry again"—the "again" implying judgment).

MARCH

MARCH 1

All things must change to something new, to something strange.
—HENRY WADSWORTH LONGFELLOW

MIRACLE MOVES

There are "miracle moves" that you can make in relationships: these are new and different ways of relating to others, and they truly are miraculous both in their simplicity and in their results. Let's take apart a miracle move that you can use. It consists of two simple actions, both grounded in this one essential concept: *Your intention creates the miracle.* If you truly *intend* to notice and wonder and create an open environment in which your partner's response can come back to you freely, without fear of judgment, your miracle move will have its intended effect. So often, though, people claim to wonder when they are merely seeking to reinforce their own perception. People claim to *notice* when they are simply *judging*. Look at the difference: To say "I notice something in your expression" is truly noticing; to say "I notice that you look angry" is to assign meaning and, likely, judgment. The same is true with wondering. To say "I wonder what you're feeling" is true wonder, whereas to say "I wonder if you're mad at me?" means that the speaker has already decided what the other is feeling and is simply seeking to reinforce it. If the response that comes back doesn't reinforce it, often the speaker will simply ignore the "incorrect" response.

■ A CONSCIOUS LIVING PRACTICE FOR TODAY ■

Having practiced noticing your partner's responses without responding, make some observations for yourself about how it changed your internal experience of the communication pattern and possible outcome. Think about how you can apply this in future conflicts and communications with your partner and with others.

Messages from the body become ignored . . . relationships suffer, becoming entanglements of lost souls wearing masks rather than dances of whole beings celebrating each other.

TEN-SECOND MIRACLES

The ten-second miracle solves two problems that you face nearly every day of your life:

- How to feel a flow of good feeling *inside* yourself, and how to open the flow when it has become dammed up.
- How to feel the flow of love and good feeling *between you and other people* you care about, and how to release its flow when it has been blocked.

■ A CONSCIOUS LIVING PRACTICE FOR TODAY ■

Close your eyes and visualize a place where you have felt happy, free. Breathe deeply and slowly, allowing good feeling to fill you to overflowing with joy. Honor that joy by not timing yourself, by not rushing. Just enjoy. This is how you can experience life day by day, hour by hour, minute by minute . . . and miraculous second by miraculous second.

....

MARCH 3

To see a World in a grain of sand,
And a Heaven in a wild flower . . . —WILLIAM BLAKE

LOOKING AND SEEING

The first step in creating miracles is "looking and seeing," which contrasts with "ignoring." By not ignoring the obvious, you put yourself squarely in touch with another's reality and with reality itself. When you do this, others see you as safe; the person who is in touch with reality is always much more safe than the person who is not. For many of you, childhood was a time of "feeling denial" and "reality twisting," when adults told you that you didn't feel what you knew you felt and when you were sometimes shamed for your honest, heartfelt way of experiencing life.

Once at a scary movie, I squirmed with discomfort, but not because of what was on the screen. A father behind me was telling his scared little boy, "You're not afraid, you're not afraid." The father said, "Just hold your breath and you'll be okay." I realized I was hearing the actual programming of a human being not to feel. Hundreds of times in therapy I'd helped people learn to feel again by doing the exact opposite of this father's counsel. "Let yourself feel," I would tell my clients, "and take a few breaths to let yourself feel safe."

■ A CONSCIOUS LIVING PRACTICE FOR TODAY ■

Having practiced being aware of the changes in affect (facial expression) you notice as you communicate with others, try practicing out loud in a few interactions today. All you will practice today is looking and wondering; for now, try using the sentence below. Keep your tone neutral and without judgment.

Say "I notice something in your expression," then relax until the person responds.

....

MARCH 4

Celebrate your existence! —WILLIAM BLAKE

WONDER LANGUAGE

The first move in creating miracles is looking around and inside yourself with curiosity. The second move is learning to express yourself in "wonder language" rather than in the language of judging or proving.

Contrast the feeling of wondering with the feeling of "thinking you know." They are completely different states of consciousness. We may see an expression on someone's face and immediately jump to "thinking we know" what the expression means. Thinking we know is always risky business, because it's heavily flavored by our own moods and prejudices.

Even though I've spent half my life honing my ability to read body language, I make mistakes all the time in my personal relationships. The other day my wife gave me a look that I interpreted as disapproval. Only after a few uncomfortable interchanges did I come to find out she was discovering a broken tooth with her tongue. It had nothing to do with me, and "thinking I knew" what it meant not only contributed to the problem; it *was* the problem.

■ A CONSCIOUS LIVING PRACTICE FOR TODAY ■

Practice adding wonder-language to your vocabulary today. Use sentences like the ones below in your interactions, and notice the reactions to it.

"I wonder what the best choice would be right now."
"I wonder how everybody's feeling right now."
"I wonder what our most positive outcome could be?"

....

MARCH 5
Think not that thy word and thine alone must be right.—SOPHOCLES

SIGNALING INTENTIONS

With two simple sentences, you have created a safe zone in which your partner can learn. You have signaled that your intentions are not about judgment or assigning your own meaning to your partner's experience but, instead, about truly wondering what your partner is feeling and experiencing. The zone you have created is "shame free," full of pure possibility for discovery. What, then, comes next? Having done everything right, you wait for your partner to respond, and his or her response is going to be inspired by your miracle move. Before I examine a miracle response, though, I'm going to spend some time laying the groundwork, over the next few days, for just what lies behind the responses you may receive. I'm going to look at personality: where it comes from and how to reach the truest sense of yourself, your personality, what I call your essence.

■ A CONSCIOUS LIVING PRACTICE FOR TODAY ■

You have done a tremendous amount of work in the past two months. It's time to take a break, today, to celebrate your work and congratulate yourself on your focus and your commitment to conscious relationship with yourself and with others.

Find some part of your day that can be yours alone: fifteen minutes, half an hour, an hour. You've earned it. Spend that time in solitude, doing something that feeds your soul: listening to music, dancing, walking, meditating, stretching out your muscles and feeling the new learnings in your head and heart and body.

You have only one choice to make, now and always:

- to open yourself to embrace truth and its constant companion, love;
- or to withdraw from truth and love, defining yourself through contraction and resistance.

MARCH 6

An ecstasy is a thing that will not go into words; it feels like music. —MARK TWAIN

FREE AND CLEAR

As you move forward on your journey, think about feelings you had yesterday as you celebrated your work. I asked you to take some time for yourself to do something that would feed your soul. If you allowed yourself to choose wisely, you spent time yesterday in the place within yourself that I am going to talk about next: *essence.* Essence is the part of you that is free, clear and uncluttered with the learning processes of life. Think of essence as what is left when everything nonessential is removed, when persona and roles and the physical self and relationships to others are all set aside for the moment. Essence simply *is:* It is pure consciousness, with nothing added.

■ A CONSCIOUS LIVING PRACTICE FOR TODAY ■

Find a piece of classical music that appeals to you—I'm partial to *Pachelbel's Canon*—and play it as you lie comfortably, listening and visualizing your birth. Inhale and exhale deeply and imagine the moments of bliss in the womb, warmth, safety, darkness. Imagine your journey beginning and feel yourself moving toward a new life, a new experience. Freeze yourself at this moment, before birth, when you are on the threshold of something unknown, when you are still at your essence. Stay in the essence for as long as you'd like, feeling it, knowing it, loving and embracing it.

MARCH 7

Where there is great love, there are always miracles.——WILLA CATHER

THE BENEFITS OF MIRACLES

I make you the following promise: If you commit yourself fully to incorporating ten-second miracles into your life, you will gain three benefits. First, you will simplify your close relationships, the most complicated part of life for many people. Second, you will feel a specific positive feeling in your body as you integrate these miracles into your life. And finally, you will come to see that you have significantly more power than you ever imagined yourself to possess. You are the source of the miracles in your life; change is in your hands.

Perhaps you are not aware of how much of your life's pain and chaos is connected to how you are in relationship with others. But once you integrate miracles into your relationships, and thus simplify and improve those relationships, you will see and feel the positive changes at every level of your life: physical and psychic, internal and external.

■ A CONSCIOUS LIVING PRACTICE FOR TODAY ■

As a meditation, close your eyes and sit comfortably, breathing deeply in and out, as you repeat this affirmation to yourself until you experience good feeling coursing through you: *I am the source of miracles in my life.*

You make a simple internal shift and suddenly a flow of good feeling courses through you, like a welcome breeze on a still day. The off-center feeling disappears, replaced by a calm sense of well-being. This is the ten-second miracle at work.

I imagine one of the reasons people cling to their hates so stubbornly is because they sense, once hate is gone, they will be forced to deal with pain.—JAMES BALDWIN

LEARNING TO LOVE YOURSELF

Learning to Love Yourself, one of my earlier books, includes a list of basic beliefs, approaches to life and attitudes that many of you hold or have held.

- I have learned to see the world the way it isn't.
- I have done this for my own survival.
- I am now interested in much more than survival.
- I can see it the way it is. (1)
- There is nothing outside myself that can save me.
- I have everything I need inside me. (2)
- All the love I have been searching for is here within me. (3)
- I demand it from others because I am unwilling to give it to myself.
- I can give it to myself.
- My very nature is love, so there is no need to search for it, no need to work at it.
- Love is the only thing I need to change.
- I am now willing to love myself. (4)

■ A CONSCIOUS LIVING PRACTICE FOR TODAY ■

If you use a computer or typewriter, sit down at it and type the sentences above that are numbered one through four without looking at the screen or paper. If you only write by hand, write out the sentences, one to a line, keeping your eye off the paper as much as possible. When you are done, read over the sentences. Read no farther in the instructions until you have finished this work.

Find the one with the most mistakes (if done on a computer/typewriter) or the one that veers most sharply off of the lines (if handwritten). Spend a few moments wondering what this sentence means to you and why it presents difficulty to you.

....

MARCH 9

This is the true joy in life, the being used for a purpose recognized by yourself as a mighty one; the being thoroughly worn out before you are thrown on the scrap heap; the being a force of nature instead of a feverish selfish little clod of ailments and grievances complaining that the world will not devote itself to making you happy.
—GEORGE BERNARD SHAW

BEING A FORCE OF NATURE

Nature is engaged in an infinite process of creation, and you're part of it. There is no "nature" separate from "you": you're it and it's you. Take comfort and joy, then, in knowing that you're a force of nature. My grandmother was a passionate gardener. In her elder years, she often winced with pain as she stooped over to tend a tomato plant or pick a weed. Once I asked her if she wanted my help in bending over to dig some potatoes out of the ground. "No," she said. "If I didn't touch the earth every day, my arthritis would be worse than it is."

■ A CONSCIOUS LIVING PRACTICE FOR TODAY ■

Spend a few minutes today appreciating nature. If you can, take a walk or sit under a tree. If the only nature you can visit is the distant sight of a tree from your office window, take a moment to appreciate it.

I mean by this Sacrament an outward and visible sign of
an inward and spiritual grace.——THE BOOK OF COMMON PRAYER

THE MEGA-RULE OF RELATIONSHIPS

The mega-rule: Relationships flourish or wither in ten-second windows of communication. Every truly important relationship communication takes less than ten seconds. Your power and well-being flow from initiating the ten-second communications, not from waiting for them to happen. Change is not carried on the wind; it is something you create from your need. The miracle steps—recognizing your ten-second windows and making miracle moves in response—are within you already; simply let yourself know them and use them.

I will continue to discuss this mega-rule and show you examples, but for now, simply take in the idea and allow yourself to wonder at the possibility that what has seemed so complicated might, in fact, be amazingly simple.

■ A CONSCIOUS LIVING PRACTICE FOR TODAY ■

Think about your most significant adult-adult relationship. Wonder about one thing that you need more of in this relationship. Do not worry about how to get it or whether you believe you deserve it or any of the other obstacles that you may set up for yourself. Just identify and let yourself feel your need.

Think to yourself about

• Which relationship you want to consider.
• The need in the relationship.

To change your life: start immediately;
do it flamboyantly; no exceptions.—WILLIAM JAMES

IN PRAISE OF FLAMBOYANCE

You're here to live out loud. One of the greatest sources of pain and suffering on this planet is the pain of unrealized potential. Many of you hang back from living out your dreams, hindered by those who specialize in squelching potential (which, of course, is usually because they aren't living out their own potential).

I recall meeting a woman of sixty-seven in a Paris park some years ago. She told me she had just walked up from Portugal, taking six weeks to do so. Furthermore, she said she'd been on the road since her retirement at sixty-two. She was walking around the world, she said, proudly showing me her eleventh pair of sneakers! Noticing her wedding ring, I asked her where her husband was. She reckoned he was probably back in Arizona watching TV. She said she'd asked him to come, but he said he didn't want to.

That's flamboyance in action.

■ A CONSCIOUS LIVING PRACTICE FOR TODAY ■

Pause for a moment to answer these questions: What, for you, would represent you at your most flamboyantly positive life? What would you be doing if you were living at your full-out best? If you knew you could not fail, what would you do differently?

MARCH 12

Thunder is good, thunder is impressive; but it is lightning that does the work.

—MARK TWAIN

AN ESSENTIAL PROBLEM, AN ESSENTIAL SOLUTION

An essential problem of conscious living is resisting love and positive energy. You resist love and positive energy because they are powerful forces that take you beyond yourself, into the unfamiliar terrain of the unknown. Also, you have often experienced traumas as a result of opening up to powerful forces, such as early sexual energy. The key transformational move is learning to accept and resonate with more positive energy. This is always a challenge, because "more positive energy" means you haven't been there before. There is a scene from an Indiana Jones movie that fits the traditional definition of a catch-22, and yet also can be viewed through my framework as an opportunity to not resist the universe. In the scene, the foothold that Indiana's foot is seeking doesn't appear *until* he makes the commitment and steps with his foot. You can see how a traditional way of experiencing this might be "damned if you do (step and perhaps fall) and damned if you don't (don't take the step and suffer some other negative consequence). I believe that making the commitment is always the solution to the problem. You increase your thermostat setting, and step into the unknown again.

■ A CONSCIOUS LIVING PRACTICE FOR TODAY ■

Make a commitment out loud—to a mirror if you are alone, or to someone else if you are accompanied. Say, "I commit this day to opening to more positive energy. I choose the daily increase of love and positive energy as a central focus of my life."

After making the commitment, take a few celebratory breaths into places that feel as though they aren't fully participating with your breath. Enjoy increasing your positive energy through the vehicle of your breathing.

....

MARCH 13

Entanglement begins the moment you step out of an equal relationship with your partner and become an advocate for your victimhood.

BE CAREFUL WHAT YOU WISH FOR

Not long ago, Laura was among three finalists for two tenure-track faculty positions and wanted the job perhaps more than she'd ever wanted *any* job. The interview and a teaching demonstration went beautifully, and since there were only three candidates for two positions, and since she was the only one of the candidates with a publishing contract for a book in the field, she felt good about her chances. After several weeks, she was told she hadn't gotten the job. She listened, nearly numb, as the department chair gave her the information. That night, she told her mother that she'd like to just crawl into bed for a day of self-pity, tending to her emotional wounds, but she couldn't take the time to do so. Still, she mused, she wished there was some built-in societal recognition of the need to take the time to grieve; her sense of loss and disappointment was significant.

Laura writes: The next day, I woke up as sick as a big dog, as we used to say in grad school. I had the highest fever I'd had since childhood, 103 degrees, and every muscle in my body—many I hadn't even known myself to possess—ached. A nasty cough had started, and my head was pounding. There was no way I was getting out of bed; I tried and nearly fell over from dizziness. Lying in bed that day, feeling beaten down by the flu and betrayed by my body, it occurred to me that my mind and body had held a meeting sometime during the night while I slept and conspired against me. My mother called and, hearing I was ill, chuckled kindly. "Be careful what you wish for, for you may surely get it," she said gently. Her words started the thought going: Had my mind and body conspired *for* me? I was, after all, getting all the time I needed to hide under the covers with my sadness.

Sometimes, you are your own worst enemy, and sometimes, you are your own best friend. It's all a matter of perspective.

■ A CONSCIOUS LIVING PRACTICE FOR TODAY ■

Tune in to your body. Focus on any areas that call themselves to your attention as you tune in. As you become aware of any aches or pains or tightness in your body, think about your emotional state right now. I'm willing to bet there's a connection. Rub the aching body part, and begin to release the emotional tightness; release the emotional tightness, and feel your body respond in kind.

....

MARCH 14

Why then, do you walk as though you had swallowed a ramrod?—EPICTETUS

SOFT IN THE MIDDLE

How do you feel about your physical self? Are you happy with your body? Many people are not; in fact, I'd venture to say that *most* people are not pleased with the body in which they live. If you hated your hometown as much as you hated the physical home of your body, wouldn't you somehow change something, even move? Why is it that you allow yourself to stay stuck in such ongoing discomfort in your body?

You live in a body-conscious society, in which the current standard for attractiveness, which varies from year to year, is nearly always unattainable without an airbrush.

Laura writes: I was having an important picture taken, and had my hair put up first. The hairdresser mentioned that he did lots of advertising work, and he let me in on a trade secret: The hair on the back of a model's head is often not styled at all. He explained that he was only concerned with what would show on camera, and so he might just clip or pin back any excess hair in the back.

"It's all a big illusion, that beauty is casual and effortless," he said. "There's a team of us standing there, right out of camera's range, waiting to reassemble the model at any second. She's sprayed and pinned and clipped and shellacked, but it's all artful; it's all to make it look like she just threw herself together."

"I wonder why we believe it, then?" I mused, but I knew the answer. We want to believe in the idea of accessible and easy perfection, and we want to believe that we, too, can look like *that*. Unless you have a team at the ready, though, you can't.

What if you redefined beauty? What if a woman sweating after a workout, a man with tears in his eyes at the sight of something touching, a young girl talking tough or a young boy talking tender, clothes of comfort rather than clothes of status or display, clean, shining skin rather than a layer of makeup hiding you from the world signified an inner beauty that has made its way outward, allowing you to live in comfort?

■ A CONSCIOUS LIVING PRACTICE FOR TODAY ■

Think about what beauty is to you. When do you feel most attractive? What kinds of clothing are you wearing? What are you doing? Make a commitment to yourself to begin to merge your inner experience of conscious living with the outward symbols of beauty in your life. Conscious beauty. What a concept!

*We only become what we are by the radical and deep-seated refusal of
that which others have made of us.*——JEAN-PAUL SARTRE

CHOICE AND CONTROL

Say the word *choice* and you're likely to elicit any number of varying
responses. There are those who are considered to have what is called an
"external locus of control." These people believe they have little effect
on the events that occur around and to them; like driftwood, they are
buffeted by the sea, washed up on the shore, carried out on another random wave, all without any doing or any control on their part. The other
group of people—and if you're reading this book and haven't tossed it
off a balcony yet, I'm betting you're in this second group—have what is
called an "internal locus of control." Not only do they know that they
influence much of what happens in their lives, but they also realize that
they are responsible for it. This is not to say that there are not random
events that occur over which you have little, if any control, but the bulk
of the things that happen to you happen because of you. Your locus of
control will have much to do with the success of your journey toward
conscious relationships. The choices you make will determine the satisfaction you feel in your heart and in your relational life.

■ A CONSCIOUS LIVING PRACTICE FOR TODAY ■

Spend a few quiet moments now playing a word association game
with yourself. As you look at each word below, notice the first word that
comes to mind for you. Give yourself time to wonder about the associ-
ations you hold.

- Choice
- Control
- Fate
- Destiny

One inch of joy surmounts of grief a span, because to laugh is proper to the man.
—FRANÇOIS RABELAIS

JOY AND LAUGHTER

Think about this: What if, instead of unearthing pain and buried hurts and anxieties when you take your first steps down the path toward a conscious relationship, you find joy and laughter? Would that be all right with you, or are you someone who knows in your gut that relationship is supposed to be hard: hard work, hard communication, hard thought, hard feeling? If so, I am about to disappoint you, because although there is work involved—as I believe there is with most worthwhile things—the main component of a conscious relationship (and, indeed, of a conscious life as a whole) is pure, deep, joyful, exuberant fun! I have known more joy telling the truth in relationships than I could ever have imagined possible. I see both the sadness and the humor as I think about a couple sitting at a nearby table at a restaurant recently. They never spoke to each other, but the woman watched my wife and me with narrowed eyes as we laughed throughout the several-hour dinner. As the woman was leaving, her husband already well ahead of her, she stopped at the table and shook her head: "I've been watching you for an hour now, and I can see you're married," she said, nodding toward our wedding rings. "I just don't see what's so *funny*." And with that, she hurried away. We grasped the connection she was trying to make between marriage and a dismal existence—and thanked ourselves and the universe that we don't live in that connection.

I have said already that there are potential pitfalls, but I also want to remind you that when you turn over the rock that hides your deepest secrets, you may be surprised to find instead of dark, damp earth a garden of paradise that contains the opportunity for bliss.

Today, observe the myriad ways you shape and shade the pure truth. Then, notice why you are shading it. For example, if you say you're hungry when you're not, do you do so to be liked? Or to be nice, to get along? Begin to notice what motivates those moments of withholding the truth.

....

MARCH 17

How old would you be if you didn't know how old you was?—SATCHEL PAIGE

THE TRUTH OF WHO YOU ARE

What would it be like to return—lovingly and gently—to the truth of who you really are? First, let fall away all the levels of identity that would have been different if you had been born and raised in a different family in a different place. Take away the religion you were brought up in, the school where you went to first grade, the town you called home. Feel inside yourself what would remain if everything had been different in your upbringing.

Early in life we leave behind the world of how we feel inside for the largely visual world of how we appear from the outside. To recover your own deep identity, let fall away the identities others have given you by their approval or disapproval. Let go of the identities you formed to please your family and the identities you formed to protect yourself from pain.

For example, you may have become a "rebel" to escape the pain of loneliness, or a "sports nut" to connect with a sports-loving parent. I know about both of these, because I used those identities. Neither of them was the real me, though. It took me many years to realize that I don't have any deep regard for sports (and certainly no talents in that area!). It was just a way to get the love and approval of my sports-obsessed grandfather, who cared about little else.

■ A CONSCIOUS LIVING PRACTICE FOR TODAY ■

Look at yourself steadily in the mirror for several minutes. As you gaze, take slow, deep breaths. Gradually let go of any layers of identity that would have been different if you'd grown up in a different family or a different place. Feel what remains.

....

MARCH 18

Man who man would be, must rule the empire of himself.——PERCY BYSSHE SHELLEY

ESSENCE AND PERSONA

By the time most of you entered your teenage years, and certainly by the time you reached adult life, you had learned to wear many personas (from the Latin word meaning "mask"). Some of the masks are to get recognition, while others are to protect you from pain. In one way, though, all of your masks are the same: They all obscure your "essence self" from your own view. Beneath all masks is the open space of essence—the "who you truly are" that is unaffected by the painful or the pleasurable experiences of life. Think of life as the light of the movie projector, while personas are the pictures flickering on the wall. The pictures serve a purpose, often giving you a glimpse into who you have been, and into who you can be. They are not the heart of you, though, nor the total of your potential. I remember Jessica Rabbit in *Who Framed Roger Rabbit?* seductively growling, "I'm not bad; I'm just drawn that way." How are you drawn? How do you draw yourself? The journey of conscious living is partly about coming to know and then befriending all your personas ... and then making your *home* in essence.

Take a moment right now to contact your essence. Relax your body and take two or three deep, slow breaths. As you do, feel the open, spacious sensation in you that has never been changed by the experiences of your life. It was there when you walked into school for the first time, and it was exactly the same the day you left. This is your essence—who you truly are.

....

MARCH 19

In a word, neither death, nor exile, nor pain, nor anything of this kind is the real cause of our doing or not doing any action, but our inward opinions and principles.
—EPICTETUS

THE COSTLY HABIT OF PROJECTION

Dropping projection can liberate a vast amount of energy in your life. Every time you project, you attribute to others something that's true for you. For example, a man may complain that his wife is too passive. Were he to own this projection, he would say "I haven't learned to be in a relationship with a powerful woman, so I require them to be passive. This must mean that I haven't opened up to my own full power. That's where the work is." Imagine how much difference this perception would make in the relationship. Projection is always born of fear. A projection is always based on the fear of fully owning the projected feeling or characteristic. The work is always in seeing the projection for what it is, then opening up to the fear that fuels it.

Think of someone you don't get along with. Picture the person's face, and get a sense of why you don't like that person. When you have a clear sense of what it is you don't like, accept that exact same quality in yourself. If it's anger you don't like about the person, embrace your own anger. If it's greed, say hello to the greedy place in yourself. As you move through your day, continue owning all the negative qualities you see outside of yourself.

....

MARCH 20

You shall see wonders.—WILLIAM SHAKESPEARE

THE THREE CIRCLES OF RELATIONSHIP

All of you live within three circles of relationship, and your lives become wonderful to the extent you keep these circles expanding. The first circle is your relationship with yourself, particularly your relationship with the creative flow inside. If you keep opening up to your creativity and expressing it in the world, your circle of connection with yourself expands, as when you toss a stone into a still pond; the more energy you put behind your action, the farther the ripples extend. The second circle is your relationship with others. Here, your circle expands when you open up to appreciate the essences of the people around you, and the ripples deepen. The third circle is your relationship with the earth and the universe. In the third circle, you are the stone, the ripple, and the pond; you are the relationship between action and reaction. When you can claim responsibility for stewardship of the earth itself and the universe as a whole, the stone carries more weight, the ripple widens past where the eye can see, and the pond deepens infinitely: the third circle expands.

When you expand the three circles, you see wonders. When you contract and shrink them, you see despair all around you and you feel it inside you.

Make a commitment to expansion in your three circles of relationship. Say to yourself or aloud, "I commit to deepening my relationship with myself, others, and the earth itself."

....

MARCH 21

What if everything turns out to be an illusion and nothing real exists? In that case, I definitely overpaid for my carpet.—WOODY ALLEN

THE JOKE THAT NEVER GETS OLD

Almost all of the happy, successful people I've ever met have an ability to laugh at themselves. One advantage of learning to laugh at yourself is that you have an endless source of entertainment at your disposal. You'll have a joke that never gets stale, because there will always be something you're doing that's amusing. You can learn just as well from laughing at your mistakes as you can from decrying them.

My wife and I have an electric teakettle we use every day. We bought it primarily because the absentminded writer my wife is married to had a habit of putting a kettle on to boil, then forgetting to take it off. The great advantage of the electric one is that it turns itself off automatically when the water has boiled. With one easy ($80) move, all our problems were solved, except . . .

The other day, deep in what Kathlyn calls my writer's trance, I went into the kitchen, filled the electric kettle with water, then proceeded to put it on the stove and turn on the gas flame under it. Before I realized my mistake, the kettle had melted down all over the burner. Faced with this mess, and the extremely unconscious action that had caused it, all I could do was laugh and start cleaning up the mess.

Kathlyn smelled the burning plastic and came into the kitchen. She took one look, laughed—bless her heart!—and started helping me clean up the mess.

Consider the alternative. I could have gotten upset, Kathlyn could have gotten upset, and we could have spent the rest of the day in blame and recrimination. Why not just laugh and clean up the mess?

■ A CONSCIOUS LIVING PRACTICE FOR TODAY ■

Set an intention today of laughing at yourself once an hour. Look for foibles to poke fun at, pomposities to puncture, mannerisms to lampoon. If you run out of ideas, ask a friend to tell you a few things about you that others find absolutely ridiculous.

....

MARCH 22

Character building begins in our infancy, and continues until death.
—ELEANOR ROOSEVELT

AUTONOMY

At the root of your beginning on this journey were twin needs: the need for unity, or connectedness with others, and the need for autonomy, or space apart from others. These are both natural, normal human needs. Why, then, are both relationship and autonomy so difficult to partake of for so many people? Let's look at autonomy first. As anyone who has spent time around a toddler knows, the stirrings toward autonomy are powerful indeed, encouraging a helpless, dependent child to try to separate from the very people who support him and give him sustenance. The human heart knows, however, that separateness is essential to psychic survival, even at the youngest age. Most of you have been wounded—many times, perhaps—in your attempts at individuation, first from your parents and then, as you grew older, from lovers. And yet you retain and even continue to fight for the sanctity of your separate self.

■ A CONSCIOUS LIVING PRACTICE FOR TODAY ■

Think back to your adolescence and try to recall a conflict that you had with your mother or father. The details are not important. All that is important for now is remembering the feelings you had at the time.

The act of withholding any aspect of yourself is fatal to a co-committed relationship.

....

MARCH 23

Awake, arise, or be forever fallen!—JOHN MILTON

BEING: A PLACE IN THE WORLD

The growth of a close adult relationship often parallels the early stages of childhood development. Your first task on earth after you are born seems simple enough: *being.* All that is required of you is that you "be," exist and receive from others. In many ways, this is sufficient in the earliest days of many new adult relationships; your partner takes great delight in you, not demanding or requesting that you do anything except exist, and you, in turn, appreciate your new partner in the same way. I am asking you to focus on this sensation of just being: breathing, existing, having your perfect place in the universe, where there is no wish for more, for less, for better or worse; you simply are, and in being, you achieve relationship with the universe that is without struggle.

Think back to the earliest days of your current or most recent intimate relationship and spend a few moments today wondering about

- The first thing I remember doing for my partner.
- The first thing I often find myself doing for partners in new relationships.
- The first memories I have of my mother or father *doing* for me.

....

MARCH 24

Teach us to give and not to count the cost.——IGNATIUS LOYOLA

DOING: A PLACE IN THE WORLD

The second task for the infant is slightly more complicated; it involves *doing*. You learn to explore and to act on and respond to the environment in rapidly evolving ways. Again, your adult relationships are similar; once the earliest rosy glow fades slightly, you may find yourself beginning to attempt to be known to your partner by doing: you cook her a complicated dinner, which tells her that you are giving and nurturing, perhaps, or maybe she challenges you to a game of basketball to illustrate that she is strong and capable and fun in multifaceted ways. Simply existing is no longer enough. In the doing stage, you are learning whether you can have connection and unity together in this relationship.

■ A CONSCIOUS LIVING PRACTICE FOR TODAY ■

Go back to the earliest days of the relationship you are in now. Can you remember the point at which you began to move from the "being" to the "doing" stages? What kinds of things did you do to make yourself known to your partner? Are these things that are naturally satisfying to you, things that you enjoy doing, or are they things that you have always done because you believe them to be of value to others or because you believe them to fit a persona that you were trying to fit? (For instance, perhaps you cooked—despite not enjoying cooking—because to be "wife material" means being able to cook). Think about how you can let yourself be known truthfully to another without falling into the trap of doing things that fit within a persona but not with who you are.

....

MARCH 25

Let there be spaces in your togetherness and let the winds of the heavens dance between you.—Kahlil Gibran

WHEN BEING AND DOING MERGE

What follows the often blissful early stages of relationship? Again, you can look toward your earliest experiences to find the answer. You simply exist, and then you begin to turn outward, to react to the world around you. Now you begin to merge the two in a significant way: you bring forth experience and feeling that is lodged in your earliest memories of being (anger, comfort, despair, and helplessness, to name a few) and merge it with your relationship with another; these can come flooding into the new and untested relationship. You have probably had the experience of looking upon your new partner and saying, "You've changed!" Maybe it happened sooner, perhaps later, but I'm willing to venture that it happened. And when these previously hidden aspects of yourself emerge, it seems blatantly obvious that they do so because of the person with whom you are in relationship.

■ A CONSCIOUS LIVING PRACTICE FOR TODAY ■

Give yourself quiet and peace for this exercise. Breathe slowly and deeply and let yourself remember your fears, as a child, of being abandoned. Perhaps you will remember a time when you were out in public with a parent and became separated, or perhaps you will remember a more permanent separation, if a parent left. Breathing deeply, let yourself again experience the fear and despair of the child whose world feels uncertain and overwhelming. Do not judge this child; love this child. Love your fear; love your despair; love your smallness in the face of such a big world.

When you deny that you are the cause of what happens to you, you tend to project it outside, on partners, bosses, the world itself. Unconscious loving thrives on victimhood.

....

MARCH 26

Understand yourself, and you will understand everything.—SHUNRYU SUZUKI

REPLICATION AND REPLACEMENT

In your earliest relationships, you mimicked what you knew from your family-of-origin relationships. For some people, that means "replication," wherein you find someone who mirrors a significant other (often a parent) from early life. For others, it means "replacement," wherein you find someone at the opposite end of the spectrum from your early significant other. Many people say, "I looked for someone who was as unlike my mother/father as I could find." Strangely enough, what they ultimately find is that the person is, by paradox, exactly like the person they were trying to avoid replicating. An example: A woman is looking for a man who is completely unlike her cold, distant, disapproving father. Instead, she finds a man who gives love glibly, almost, and who touches everyone frequently and who seems to look upon everyone with approval. Sounds good, right? Ultimately, though, the woman discovers that she feels ignored because the man is so busy spreading his love around indiscriminately; she could be anyone, she feels, and still be loved by this man. His touches mean nothing because they are also indiscriminate, and so she feels untouched. His approval is without basis—everyone is wonderful! What makes her special?

■ A CONSCIOUS LIVING PRACTICE FOR TODAY ■

I commit to knowing about my past patterns in seeking others for relationship.

I commit to looking at my patterns of replicating and replacing in relationship.

I commit to choosing a path that meets my adult needs rather than childhood needs.

I commit to having love and to being responsible for finding and growing that love.

A healthier relationship becomes possible only when both people are willing to base their actions on the knowledge that they are the source of their reality.

....

MARCH 27

Consistency is the last refuge of the unimaginative.—Oscar Wilde

WHEN TO LEAVE AND WHEN TO STAY

I have discussed the need for unity and for autonomy in relationships in terms of its formation of the relationship: how you seek out a lover, how you approach early relationships. What about when relationships end, though? In your earliest relationships, how do you know when it's time to leave and how do you know how to leave or be left? Again, you trace the lines of your history, your heart. Those lines can tell you much about not only where you have been, but also about where you are now—and where you will be ten years from now if you make no changes. Have you ever found yourself in a relationship or a job, perhaps, that consisted mainly of misery, and suddenly found yourself thinking of the future? The thought often goes like this: I will not look back at my life in ten years . . . and still be here, in this. My life will not turn out this way.

The most significant factor at play as relationships draw to a close or change in status is projection. Simply, projection is the act of putting the responsibility for your own thoughts and feelings and behaviors on another. I feel angry and so I begin to notice that you seem short-tempered, and I accuse you of being angry. But why would you do this? Self-protection. In the short term, isn't it often easier to blame than to wonder, to point the finger of self-righteousness rather than to sit with your own weaknesses?

■ A CONSCIOUS LIVING PRACTICE FOR TODAY ■

Give yourself some time today to think on these thoughts:

- I knew my first love relationship was going to end when _____.
- When the relationship ended, I felt _____.
- I think that I felt this way because it mirrored _____.

Learning to perceive the truth within yourself and speak it clearly to others is a delicate skill.

....

MARCH 28

No pleasure is comparable to the standing upon the vantage-ground of truth.
—FRANCIS BACON

TRYING ON THE TRUTH

It is somewhat simpler to think of yourself as a person who embraces self-knowledge than it is to practice the art of complete honesty. You start with yourself before you begin with others, just as you might first try on a new expression or a daring piece of clothing in privacy; you take the tentative first steps toward telling the complete truth in the privacy of your heart. This is not easy; you are often adept at hiding, at subterfuge, even with yourself. Perhaps especially with yourself.

Be gentle with yourself when you first try on the truth. Don't force yourself into things that don't yet fit, but don't drape yourself with things that are too large for you, either. Neither will serve you. Instead, breathe in patience and self-love as you allow yourself to gradually come to know what is true—and what is not—for you and of you and in you.

■ A CONSCIOUS LIVING PRACTICE FOR TODAY ■

Recall a time when you said something, as a child, that resulted in negative responses from adults around you. This may be a memory that you have only through family lore, but put yourself into the memory and search for these answers:

- In my memory, I said _____.
- This must have made me feel _____.
- Before I tell a difficult truth now, I feel _____.

MARCH 29

Reason is not measured by size or height, but by principle.—EPICTETUS

BECOMING A PRODUCER AND A DISTRIBUTOR

Many of you keep yourself trapped in a cycle of negativity by approaching life with a "What's in it for me?" mentality. This way of looking at the world puts you in a consumer mode that, paradoxically, guarantees that you will always experience a lack. In other words, in love as well as in money, the urge to get what you can dooms you to scarcity, because it presumes you don't have enough. People have turned their lives around in an eyeblink by realizing that they can produce love rather than demand it from others.

In therapy, a woman was complaining that her husband didn't give her the love and attention she craved. "That may be true," I said, "but let's start by focusing on the way you pay attention to you. When's the last time you sat still for a minute and paid loving attention to yourself?" She admitted she had never done it for even a second. "Then do it now," I said. We sat together for a silent minute, simply paying loving attention to ourselves. This minute stretched on to another and another. Finally she opened her eyes and smiled. "I see what you mean. There wasn't any room for him to pay me the kind of attention I wanted." She had just discovered the power of taking over the producer role rather than staying locked in the consumer mode.

■ A CONSCIOUS LIVING PRACTICE FOR TODAY ■

Take a few breaths—slow, deep breaths. As you breathe in, feel yourself connecting to the source of all energy. As you breathe out, feel yourself contributing to abundance in the world. Breathing in . . . celebrating your connection to the source. . . . Breathing out . . . celebrating your contribution to life. Pause several times during the day to enjoy this type of breathing.

....

MARCH 30

It is not because things are difficult that we do not dare;
it is because we do not dare that they are difficult.—SENECA

BEING PRESENT IN YOUR BODY

Basic body awareness is an important conscious living skill, one at which we could all use more practice. If you had spent an hour a day—

from first grade through high school—learning to be aware of your body and celebrating it as the miracle it is, you probably would not want to abuse it with drugs, overeating, and overstressing yourself. Body awareness means that you can do simple but powerful things such as

- Notice where you feel the flow of life energy and where you don't.
- Appreciate the subtle difference between various emotions such as fear, anger, sadness, and longing.
- Distinguish the difference between hunger and loneliness, for example, so that you would not eat when you're lonely.
- Be able to relax your body organically, through deep breathing or other means, so that you can manage stressful situations.

■ A CONSCIOUS LIVING PRACTICE FOR TODAY ■

Take ten seconds right now to scan your body with your awareness. Simply feel and sense. There are no right answers; just listen and learn what there is to learn. As you move through the day today, pause occasionally to tune in to your body sensations—for no reason except the pure joy of awareness.

....

MARCH 31

Thus in the beginning the world was so made that certain signs come before certain events.—CICERO

GOING TO THE RIGHT STORE

If you know you want grapefruit, says an ancient therapists' axiom, don't go shopping for it in a shoe store. The same thing holds true in looking for acknowledgment and recognition. Part of the art of getting acknowledgment is knowing you deserve it. Another part of the art is being smart about where you go for it. If you know a particular friend or family member is stingy with appreciation, don't bother complaining when they don't appreciate you. Just look for another store and go shopping there.

■ A CONSCIOUS LIVING PRACTICE FOR TODAY ■

Make a list, on paper or in your mind, of several people you can rely on for acknowledgment. These people genuinely appreciate your being in the world, and will tell you so easefully. These are not people you have to wring appreciation out of. When you have your list, make a point today of appreciating them for appreciating you. Call them or drop them a note of appreciation.

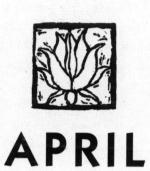

APRIL

APRIL 1

Don't find fault—find a remedy.—HENRY FORD

TURN COMPLAINTS INTO REQUESTS OR ACTION

One of the most powerful moves you can make in your year of conscious living is learning to turn your complaints into requests or action. Think about it for a moment: If every ounce of energy human beings use in complaining was dedicated to productive change, we could clear up many of the world's problems virtually overnight. It takes courage to turn a complaint into a request or effective action. It requires that you think about what needs to be done rather than about what wasn't done. It requires that you get outside the negative-thinking cycle of "What's wrong with me? What's wrong with you? What's wrong with the world?" and make a courageous leap of thought to "Forget what's wrong—let's focus on what needs to be done."

■ A CONSCIOUS LIVING PRACTICE FOR TODAY ■

Think about some of the complaints you've voiced recently. Were they complaints about yourself? Or were they complaints about other people? The world itself? Focusing on two or three key complaints, shift them to action steps or requests. For example, if one of your complaints is the quality of a road you drive on, write a note to the highway department requesting that it be fixed (or else enjoy the bumpy ride).

*Everything that irritates us about others can lead us to
an understanding of ourselves.*—CARL G. JUNG

PROJECTION

Why would you project onto others your own feelings, thoughts, and behaviors? For many of you, it seems easier to stay locked in power struggles with others than to look into the true source of the struggle within yourself. Surely it is easier to blame another—and surely these feelings weren't here before she or he came along, right? Allow yourself to remember that they were indeed here, and in great abundance, before this relationship began. They were there—in their earliest formation—when your parents cradled you as an infant, and they were there when you had your first teenaged love attachment, and they are here now. They are yours to claim, to examine with wonder, to love. Why love something so hidden and dark and shameful? Don't rush to judgment so easily, for projection gives you the possibility of change. Without it, you would have a hard time seeing your hidden self. By opening your eyes and your heart and your mind to the repetitive patterns in a close relationship, you allow your hidden self to come to light. If you pay close attention to these patterns, you will readily see the areas in yourself that require fine-tuning or a major overhaul.

■ A CONSCIOUS LIVING PRACTICE FOR TODAY ■

Choose two significant intimate relationships of your life, one past and one present, and identify several character traits for each person with whom you had that relationship:

See any similarities? Any patterns in the types of significant others you tend to choose? Look deeper if not. Remember that sometimes opposites are identical twins in terms of behavioral results.

APRIL 3

Believe not your own brother—believe, instead,
your own blind eye.—RUSSIAN PROVERB

ACCEPTING FEELINGS

I have found that there are three things that people do to entrench themselves more deeply in relationship ruts. Thousands of times, working with couples in therapy, I have seen the fallout caused by *not accepting feelings, not telling the truth, and not keeping agreements.* By turning these three practices into their positive opposites, you create three powerful strategies for successful relationships. Let's talk first about accepting feelings, both your own and the feelings of others. When you do not allow yourself to know and experience your feelings, you put yourself into a state of conflict. The same is true when you do not allow others to feel what they feel in relation to you. Laura writes: As in my encounter with the monsters, when I told my son, in essence, that he did not know what he felt, any interaction in which feeling—an unarguable truth—is denied is an interaction that is damaging to both people involved.

■ A CONSCIOUS LIVING PRACTICE FOR TODAY ■

Answer this question for yourself:

At this moment I feel _____.

Whatever you are feeling at this moment—happy, distracted, frustrated, calm—let yourself know it fully. Think of other times when you have had similar feelings and see if there is a connection. Let it link to your body. How do your physical sensations mirror the emotional experience? Sit with the feeling; embrace it because it is yours; love it.

When it is time for you to resolve a particular issue in your life, lasso someone to work it out with.

I'm armed with more than complete steel—the justice of my quarrel.
—CHRISTOPHER MARLOWE

TELLING THE TRUTH

The second powerful strategy in successful relationships is telling the truth. The very idea appears subversive and dangerous to many people. What I hear, time and again, is that people are afraid that if they tell the truth they will cause hurt to their partners. I believe that this fear masks the real fear: that many people do not want to have to deal with their partner's reaction when they tell the truth. It seems that many people prefer the deadness of ritualized truth-hiding in their relationships to the raw, electric aliveness that telling the truth produces. It seems obvious to me that if you tell the truth you have a relationship; if you don't, you don't. A relationship is between two equals who tell the truth to each other, not between two people who hide themselves and, perhaps, protect the other. Dalma Heyn, in her wonderful book *Marriage Shock*, talks about women hiding expensive clothing purchases from their husbands. Each woman insists that she is not lying and that her husband would not object, but each also (initially) insists that she is protecting her husband. As they explore the issue further, the absurdity becomes clear: they are protecting their husbands from what? The knowledge that women's clothing is expensive? The knowledge that their wives were in a store? What could be such a big secret as to require a lie? Heyn's thesis supports my contention: These women are protecting *themselves*, not from disapproval from their husbands but from their own disapproving voices, voices that say, you're self-indulgent; you're too free with money; you're this; you're that. Lies are self-protection; make no mistake about it.

Think of a lie you have told. Now think of a time you have pretended recently. When you consider the "lie" and the "pretense," think about two things for each:

Who you told yourself you were protecting.
Who was ultimately harmed.

Are they really so different? Look carefully within yourself to be certain that those pretenses you excuse are not simply glorified lies. Who, after all, are you protecting? And are you so fragile as to really need such protection?

....

APRIL 5

What lies behind us and what lies before us are small matters compared to what lies within us.—RALPH WALDO EMERSON

KEEPING AGREEMENTS

I have discussed feeling all of your feelings and I have discussed honesty. What about breaking agreements? I'm thinking about a young friend whose parents divorced when he was still a toddler. He lived with his mother, a faithful and steady friend. His father, an exciting but shiftless man, would occasionally roar into the boy's life on a motorcycle, showering him with gifts that were expensive and useless, totally out of synch with the boy's age and life. When the rare weekends approached that the boy's father was coming for a visit, he would be excited, barely able to eat or sleep. Hours would tick by, and often the father would not show up. His mother would try to soften the blow, but my young friend's heart was broken. This happened countless times, and I watch him now as he breaks agreement after agreement in his own adult relationships. It is not inevitable that you will repeat the patterns of your early life, but it requires conscious attention and commitment to ensure that you don't. Agreements, whether to yourself or to others, should not be made if they cannot, or will not, be honored. You have the strength and the intelligence and the heart to know what you are willing and not willing to do. Allow yourself to know the difference and commit yourself to keeping your agreements; then watch your heart and your relationships blossom with the joy that trust, the result of kept agreements, brings.

■ A CONSCIOUS LIVING PRACTICE FOR TODAY ■

Commitment: *I commit to examine my heart before I make commitments, and to ask myself:*

- Is this something I choose to do?
- Is this something I need to do?
- Is this something I will carry through with?
- How will I damage myself and others if I do not keep this agreement?

Commitment: *I commit to keeping the agreements I make, and to not making those commitments that I will not keep.*

....

APRIL 6

Perfection is finally attained, not when there is no longer anything to add, but when there is no longer anything to take away.—ANTOINE DE SAINT-EXUPÉRY

THE RELATIONSHIP YOU WANT

You are setting the stage for performing miracles in your life. I have started by discussing some of the dynamics that exist in adult relationships and by asking you to examine the ways in which you lay claim to these dynamics. Woven throughout is a discussion of the process of creating miracles, but I am moving slowly on purpose, because there is much work that can be done along the path toward having the relationship that you want with yourself and with others. Sometimes I ask you to look at the underpinnings to what you do, and sometimes I ask you to practice new behaviors with yourself and with others, but every day on this journey there is one constant: I am with you and wishing only the best for you in loving and being loved.

■ A CONSCIOUS LIVING PRACTICE FOR TODAY ■

When it comes to love, what is the best for you? I can wish it for you, but I cannot tell you what it is; that is up to you. With today's exercise, you will begin a practice you will return to throughout this year. It is the practice of mission- and goal-setting, a practice I borrowed from corporate work. Today's step is simply to repeat this affirmation to yourself: *I know what is best for me and I will see that I get it.*

You shape the course of your life by moments in which you open to intimacy or shrink away from it.

....

APRIL 7

The great thing in this world is not so much where we stand, as in what direction we are moving.—OLIVER WENDELL HOLMES

PAIN AND PURPOSE

Let's talk today about pain and the role it plays in your life. In humanity's distant past, poets and philosophers may have talked about emotional pain, but the average person did not. That concept was reserved for the physical self, so let's start there. Pain is generally viewed by scientists who study physical issues as the body's method of alerting you to trouble. Your belly sends sharp pains shooting forth, and it is discovered that your appendix is diseased and preparing to rupture;

without the signal of pain, the rupture would occur unnoticed, followed by sepsis, followed by death. Pain warns you not to touch hot objects like stoves and not to bend your body into certain positions; it also warns you that you *should* do certain things—you have pain that goes away, perhaps, from stretching or breathing well or quitting smoking. Psychic pain serves the same role. That lonely ache goes away when you stretch your life to include others; that sharp misery ceases when you let go of or change a toxic relationship. The key is learning to make the right choices at critical junctures in life; learn this skill and you can eliminate most pain from your life.

■ A CONSCIOUS LIVING PRACTICE FOR TODAY ■

Close your eyes and spend a few moments today visualizing pain you have felt, both physical and psychic or emotional. Ask yourself these questions as you feel how you experience pain:

When I think of pain I see the color _____.
When I feel physical pain it often settles in my _____.
When I feel psychic pain it often settles in my _____.
To eliminate psychic pain my practice has been to _____.

All too often we use the opportunities for growth as justifications for holding more tenaciously to our old positions, the positions that do not bring happiness but are simply familiar.

APRIL 8

First say to yourself what you would be, and then do what you have to do.—EPICTETUS

PERFECTION

I hope you're learning not to be a perfectionist. The more I've lightened up on my perfectionism over the years, the more fun I've had and the more effective my actions have become. The only times I seem to do things perfectly is when I'm not thinking about doing them perfectly at all. I played a round of golf on vacation a while back, and I happened to be blessed with a partner who was a relentless perfectionist. With every shot, he groaned, cursed, critiqued, and cajoled his ball, his swing, his club, and the course. I don't think he experienced a moment of joy all afternoon. He gave me a model of what I most do not want to be, on the golf course or anywhere else in life.

I've learned to approach my infrequent rounds of golf—and my frequent rounds of life—in a completely different way. For me, it's a walk in a beautiful park, enriched with a light purpose. For me, the joy of golf is in the feeling of the swing, the sound of the ball-strike, the flight of the ball, the beauty of the surroundings. My partner apparently reserved his joy for the perfect outcome, and it just never happened.

■ A CONSCIOUS LIVING PRACTICE FOR TODAY ■

Pause for a moment to circulate this thought through your mind: I'm not perfect; I'm fully human and fully flawed. I allow myself to make plenty of mistakes and learn from my experiences.

All our interior world is reality . . . and that perhaps more so
than our apparent world.—MARC CHAGALL

EMBRACING ESSENCE

You can visualize and embrace essence as who you were in your original form, as a pure, loving heart not yet bombarded with the world's messages: *Be safe! Take care! Don't feel too much! Be this! Do that!* (Try hanging around the parent of a toddler for an hour or so—for that matter, try *being* the parent of a toddler for an hour or so—and you'll see what I mean! The messages come early and they come in hordes.)

It can be hard work, separating who you are now from who you might have been, except for one saving grace: your essence is not lost. It is still inside of you awaiting a signal from you that it is welcome to blossom—*more* than welcome; indeed, you will embrace it with all the joy and ecstasy of a parent embracing a longed-for newborn for the first time. Words, as Mark Twain says, are not adequate, and so you will dwell in the realm of feeling, of music, of the soul, as you begin to reclaim your birthright: your essence.

■ A CONSCIOUS LIVING PRACTICE FOR TODAY ■

The next time you have the opportunity to hold a very young baby, do so, and feel the ways in which this new person is completely of and in essence. Breathe deeply of the infant's unique scent, and feel the incredible softness of his or her skin. Listen to the sounds of deep breathing the infant makes; babies know, instinctively, how to breathe well. This infant that you hold is nothing less than pure essence. Learn something as you hold this bundle of essence: learn how to allow yourself to become more of who you are, and less of who you are supposed to be.

APRIL 10

Self-command is the main elegance.—RALPH WALDO EMERSON

A FORCE-FIELD OF ENERGY

Your essence is your core, your body, and over it, as you grow, you learn to drape personas, the clothing that hides your true self. I recall, on seeing my wife, Kathlyn, for the first time, being aware of an energy that surrounded her, a powerful force-field of essence. When I looked at her more closely, I also noticed her clothing, the type that has always appealed to me most—bright colors, flowing fabrics—and I was aware that there was no persona; Kathlyn's essence and her outer self were one and the same, which is undoubtedly why I responded to her so power-fully. But for many people, there is a huge disparity between the outer persona (worker, parent, child, spouse) and the inner essence. As these people slip in and out of various personas, sometimes they experience the occasional sense of confusion and dissonance as they wonder, "Whatever happened to *me*? Who am I? Where did I go?" Others, having let their essence become swallowed up in the roles of life, which are worn heavily, like crosses, never even ask the fundamental questions about their existence.

■ A CONSCIOUS LIVING PRACTICE FOR TODAY ■

Identify several key personas in your life. These may be roles that you play (i.e., "daughter") or they may be a collection of character traits that make up a role (i.e., "dutiful daughter"). Do not judge these roles (personas often serve a very useful purpose!); your work today is simply to get to know your various personas.

Essence has a way of growing even from humble beginnings when there is a willingness to make commitments and live authentically.

I am on the side of the unregenerate who affirm the worth of life as an end in itself, as against the saints who deny it.—OLIVER WENDELL HOLMES

FIGHT OR FLIGHT

You are probably familiar with the psychological theory of "fight or flight." Going back to when humans were fighting off all manner of dangerous creatures, our bodies developed two responses to threat. The first is to fight against the foe, to try to defeat it and emerge the victor, in control. The second is to flee from the enemy. In modern times, your body—and your mind—still experiences these physiological responses when there is perceived threat, and even when that threat is from emotional issues that have come to feel like the wild forest beasts that once endangered us. I propose another response, a third option: flow. Don't fight or flee; flow. In other words, tune in to the feelings and be with them until they pass. Strong feelings, like thunderstorms, have a beginning, a middle—and an end. They may gather within you ominously and rage during the worst of the storm, but they will not last indefinitely. You can ride them out.

■ A CONSCIOUS LIVING PRACTICE FOR TODAY ■

Talk or think yourself through the following thoughts:

The feeling that I experience in my life that is most threatening to me is the feeling of _____. I can tell that the storm of feeling is gathering strength because my body _____ and because my thoughts _____. I can tell when I'm in the strongest part of the storm because I feel _____ and I _____. My body signals me that the storm is ending by _____ and _____. I promise myself that I will begin to focus on the stages of my emotional storms and that I will practice the art of flowing, instead of fighting or fleeing, allowing myself to ride out the storm and to embrace my own powerful feelings.

To claim your full birthright as a human being, you need to claim your ability to be with whatever is there. Otherwise, you are a human fleeing.

....

Whatsoever ye have spoken in darkness shall be heard in the light;
and that which ye have spoken in the ear in closets
shall be proclaimed upon the housetops.—LUKE 12:13

PERSONAS

Why, if personas cause so much pain and backward movement, would you cling to them so desperately? For a number of reasons. The persona often garners external rewards. A "good mother," for instance, is rewarded with a society that approves of her, children who respond to her, and a sense that she is being what society has asked her to be and what at least a part of her wishes to be. The dark side, however, is far more complicated: the good mother may also be rewarded by a sense of moral superiority; by her sacrifice, for instance, she is right and others are wrong. The persona may also serve as a way of avoiding frightening, overwhelming feelings, perhaps the good mother's feelings of rage at having given up her dreams, say, to become an artist, or her powerful unmet needs for solitude. Personas allow you to avoid such feelings and to corner the market on superiority. That's a powerful combination for some and a distancing combination for all.

■ A CONSCIOUS LIVING PRACTICE FOR TODAY ■

Look back at the personas you identified on April 10. Today, spend some time identifying external and internal rewards that you have frequently received for each persona.

APRIL 13

What you see in others has more to do with who you are than who other people are.

—EPICTETUS

PROJECTIONS AND PERSONAS

Personas—the masks you wear to protect yourself from pain and to get the recognition of others—keep you from feeling the clarity and open spaciousness of who you are at the core. When you cling to a persona, it shapes the way you see the world.

For example, if I walk into a party wearing my "approval seeker" persona, I will see others at the party as "people to be pleased." If I'm wearing a "misunderstood genius" persona, the room is full of people who probably won't understand my genius. In other words, we project an image of our personas onto other people. No wonder we have so much trouble connecting with them.

■ A CONSCIOUS LIVING PRACTICE FOR TODAY ■

Think of a past relationship that didn't work very well. Ask yourself: What was I seeing in the other person that was really a projection of a part of me I didn't like very much?

APRIL 14

No man, for any considerable time, can wear one face to himself and another to the multitude without finally getting bewildered as to which may be true.

—NATHANIEL HAWTHORNE

MASTERING PROJECTION

If your close relationships are to be successful, the problem of projection needs to be understood and mastered. Yesterday I invited you to look at a past relationship in which projection played a role. What usually happens in a relationship is that if both people are willing to let go of personas and projections, the relationship flourishes. If they aren't, it withers and dies.

From thirty years of therapy experience, I have seen one particular move produce more magic than practically any other: When you find yourself complaining about something in another person, apply the same complaint to yourself first. If I am unhappy with my partner's anger, for example, I first need to look at how I'm out of touch with my own.

Relationships flourish only when there is essence-to-essence connection—in other words, the magic of relationships occurs when the free and clear part of one person connects with the free and clear part of another.

■ A CONSCIOUS LIVING PRACTICE FOR TODAY ■

Ask yourself: What is a common complaint I have about a close relationship?

Now ask yourself: How could this complaint be applied to me?

If we approach ourselves with an attitude of humble inquiry, there are great rewards in the richness of relationship learning.

....

APRIL 15

As a man is, so he sees.——WILLIAM BLAKE

A BLANKET OF GOODS

Focus for a moment on "things," the clutter of goods with which you surround yourself. In particular, think about the role that material goods serve. If you met a man with a ragged beard and old, torn clothing standing in front of a broken shack, what judgments might you make about him, about his life? If you later saw the same man in a sweeping mansion filled with beautiful art, with a Mercedes adorning the long, curved driveway looping around the house, how would those judgments change? Might you perhaps decide that the man is eccentric, an artist maybe, someone too caught up in the throes of creation to concern himself with Armani clothing and salon haircuts? It's all in the image, of course. How important is image to you? How tightly are you sheltering your resources today? How much do you define yourself in terms of what you *have* rather than what you *are*? If you lost it all tomorrow, ask yourself what would be left. The important question: *Who are you without the blanket of goods that surrounds you?* If the answer is hard to come by, it is time to divest, time to simplify, time to build up the inner existence and let go of the outer life that has defined and hidden you.

■ A CONSCIOUS LIVING PRACTICE FOR TODAY ■

Make a list (on paper or in your head) of the three things on which you spend the most money each month (house, car, electronic equipment, etc.). Make another list of the three things that you spend time doing that bring you the most satisfaction. Compare the two lists. The more overlap, the more I would suggest you divest; if both your greatest expense and your greatest pleasure is a car, I would suggest that you are not focusing on a rich inner life but on a material outer life. And, I would wonder, from what are you running?

Simply being present with what is has so much power that you often do not give yourself more than a split second of it.

A mind not to be chang'd by place or time.
The mind is its own place,
and in itself can make a heaven of hell,
a hell of heaven.——JOHN MILTON

WHAT ARE YOU PRETENDING TO KNOW?

A bumper sticker that was popular a few years back said, "What Are You Pretending Not to Know?" That's a terrific question, one that helps lift the lid off self-delusion. But a variation of it also has a great deal of power: "What Are You Pretending to Know?" Pretending you know something stops the discovery process in its tracks. It seals a lid on a particular aspect about yourself, other people, or the world. It's easy to joke about fundamentalists who once pretended to know the world was flat or that the sun revolved around the earth. It wasn't that long ago, though, that curious people lost their lives for challenging the validity of those illusions.

■ A CONSCIOUS LIVING PRACTICE FOR TODAY ■

Take a look around your life for any places where you're pretending to know something you really ought to be celebrating as an active inquiry. Maybe you pretend you know what you can earn every year or how much love you can give and receive. When you think of a few areas, unseal the lid and turn it into an active inquiry. Wondering always feels better than knowing (especially if the knowing isn't really something you know!).

One kind word can warm three winter months.——JAPANESE PROVERB

OPPORTUNITIES FOR CONNECTION

Many of us don't appreciate that our lives are shaped by tiny moments of choice. We make hundreds of thousands of them each day, from the most mundane ("What tie shall I wear?") to the most profound ("Shall I become a parent?").

One of the most important choices we get from moment to moment is whether to reach out and connect authentically with another person or stay within the bubble of our own perceptions of that person.

Recently I met a person whom I hadn't seen in a few months. When I caught sight of her waving to me, I had a split-second realization that there was something I was angry at her about that I had not shared with her. Within a moment of saying hello, I found out she was leaving the country on a vacation. There I was, faced with a choice. Should I take advantage of the opportunity life had afforded me, to communicate with her and tell her what had been on my mind? Or should I let it go? I made the decision to tell her, and so I did. It took just a few moments to complete the communication, and we gave each other a hug and said good-bye. As I turned to leave, I was flooded with a deep sense of appreciation for her, especially for the way she'd listened to me. I called to her and spoke my appreciation to her. She responded with an appreciation of me. I left with a warm glow in my body, and I bet she did, too.

■ A CONSCIOUS LIVING PRACTICE FOR TODAY ■

Pause for a moment to recommit to several things we've visited before. They are so important they bear focusing on again, and again.

Say, "I commit to accepting all my feelings, and to speaking about them authentically with people I meet."

If we could see the miracle of a single flower clearly, our whole life would change.
—BUDDHA

RESPONSIVE MIRACLE MOVES

There are three basic elements to a responsive miracle move: stating your feelings, claiming ownership of those feelings, and wondering about something, usually your behavior. These elements parallel the core ingredients of a conscious relationship: accepting feelings, telling the truth, and keeping agreements. The first makes a clear parallel; in a sense, stating your feelings is simply an operationalized version of accepting your feelings: it is a statement that you both know and accept your truth. The second, claiming ownership of your feelings, is truth-telling put to the test; having acknowledged that you are experiencing a certain feeling, are you willing to be honest enough with yourself and others to own what you feel, to see its place in your life? And the third, wondering, harkens back to your agreement, to committing to yourself to following the path of wonder rather than doubt.

■ A CONSCIOUS LIVING PRACTICE FOR TODAY ■

Today, your work and your play are to exist in a state of wonder. For the next twenty-four hours, focus on allowing yourself to settle into a state of wondering—about your feelings, about the behaviors you exhibit, about the relationships in which you are involved. Do not judge, do not plan, do not do anything except wonder:

- What am I feeling?
- What am I doing?
- What is in this relationship for me?

APRIL 19

From without, no wonderful effect is wrought within ourselves, unless some interior, responding wonder meets it.—HERMAN MELVILLE

BREATHING KNOWLEDGE

Take a deep breath and look at what you have learned in just a little more time spent exploring and journeying:

- You have permission to make mistakes.
- A conscious journey consists of accepting and stating your feelings.
- A conscious journey consists of telling and owning your truth.
- A conscious journey consists of a commitment to wonder.
- A conscious journey consists of a commitment to keeping agreements.
- Miracle moments are signaled by windows of feeling and windows of unfairness.
- Responding to miracle moments is simple if you state your feelings, own those feelings, and wonder about why you do and say the things you do.

I believe in moments of reflection, of taking stock of where I am, who I am, where I am going. Perhaps at this stage of your journey, it is time to step back and consider your starting point, changes you have made, and changes you feel beginning in you like new life. A wonderful way to begin to take stock is to check in with your body, allowing it to tell you what is new about you and what hangs on tenaciously, the ghosts of the past still clinging, like mist, around your heart.

■ A CONSCIOUS LIVING PRACTICE FOR TODAY ■

Read the instructions through before beginning this exercise.
Take ten deep inhalations and exhalations, allowing yourself to focus

completely on your physical sensations. Feel your belly and chest rise and fall with each breath, and let the thoughts of the day leave you with each breath until you are focused totally on your body. Allow yourself to focus in on the body part that is making itself most known to you, and caress it with your breath, encouraging it to tell you what it holds and why it is calling out to you right now. Unlock its secrets, encouraging them forth and embracing them, loving your joy, your fear, your past, all of the parts that make up who you are in this moment.

....

APRIL 20

To be seventy years young is sometimes far more cheerful and hopeful than to be forty years old.—OLIVER WENDELL HOLMES JR.

GOING BEYOND YOUR COMFORT ZONE

Some of the most vital people I've met are elders who make a practice of getting out of their comfort zone on a regular basis. At a psychology conference, I struck up a conversation with a vibrant, witty man of seventy-seven who was there to give a speech. I was impressed by his wisdom and zest for living, and I asked him point-blank how he got that way. He told me he'd been dying inside as a bored lawyer of forty-four, when suddenly the urge had come over him to become a medical doctor. When no U.S. school would take him, he learned a foreign language and went to medical school in Europe. By the time he finished his degree and residency he was fifty-one, an age when many people start looking forward to retiring. Not him, though. Having grown up in Manhattan, he was uncomfortable away from a city, so to overcome this discomfort he took a job as doctor at a remote reservation in the desert. Finally, I asked him what he was doing for fun. With a twinkle in his eye he said, "This year I'm doing ballroom dancing and learning to play sax."

As you go through your day, look for any ways in which you're living within your comfort zone. Ask yourself if there are "growth edges" you are not exploring because to do so would disturb your routines. Select a growth edge and take action on it—even if it's uncomfortable to do so.

....

APRIL 21

It is often hard to bear the tears that we ourselves have caused.—MARCEL PROUST

DISTURBANCES OF RESPONSIBILITY

I take inspiration from M. Scott Peck's thoughts about responsibility in his well-known book *The Road Less Traveled*. He says, "Mental health problems are basically disturbances of responsibility. Neurotics take too much responsibility; people with character disorders take too little." As a human, you tend to see and experience responsibility as a burden or as a restriction of your freedom, when, in fact, it is the path to wholeness and to incredible freedom and lightness.

It is exhilarating to know yourself to be wholly responsible for your life—think back to those first heady moments in which you finally felt responsible for yourself, perhaps after you finished school and began working. Wasn't everything possible? Wasn't the world rich with possibility? This was because you knew that you were at the helm, piloting your own life. A powerful and freeing experience, responsibility.

■ A CONSCIOUS LIVING PRACTICE FOR TODAY ■

Take a few moments to think about a significant intimate relationship you are currently in, or, if you are not in one at present, a recent one.

Answer these questions for yourself:

The relationship I have in mind is _____.
Our most frequent conflict is about _____.
This person at times reminds me of (another person) _____.
This conflict mirrors other conflicts I've been involved in because
   it _____.

Responsibility is a celebration of wholeness.
The corollary of dropping projection is taking full responsibility.

....

Live truth instead of expressing it.——ELBERT HUBBARD

CREATING LASTING CHANGE

The foundation of a conscious life always has been, and likely always will be, integrity. I had the pleasure of walking around the Great Pyramid a few years back, and I can say from personal experience that this structure has a great deal of integrity. It doesn't look like it's budged an inch in ages. One reason for its stability is the vast foundation of precisely cut stones, each of which is aligned in its own integrity.

Imagine your conscious life as a pyramid, with a firm foundation of integrity below and a compelling vision at the top. Many people go about it wrongside up. They have a powerful vision but don't pay attention to their integrity base. When the winds of change blow, they get caught up in the breeze without a solid support under them.

■ A CONSCIOUS LIVING PRACTICE FOR TODAY ■

Take a moment right now to inspect the integrity foundation of your life. Are there places where the foundation needs shoring up? Specifically, are there feelings you're out of touch with? Are there unspoken truths? Are there agreements you have overlooked or broken? Patch up the foundation today by handling the issue. The energy that will be freed up by doing this can literally be awesome.

....

APRIL 23

If you would be a real seeker of truth, it is necessary at least once in your life to doubt all things.—RENÉ DESCARTES

DEEP LISTENING

Many people do not listen to themselves deeply enough to know how they feel. They also do not know how to listen to their colleagues deeply enough to draw the best thinking out of them. It took me a long time to figure out that how I listened to people determined how they spoke to me. I used to complain that people didn't tell me the truth in my close relationships, but then I realized I listened to practically everyone through a judgmental filter. If people do not feel that they can be heard without judgment, they will not speak the truth. A key listening skill is how you listen to yourself, particularly to your feelings. Many of you listen and speak to yourself highly critically, as if bent on finding fault with yourself. A better way to listen to yourself (and others) is with a generous, open heart in which you experience freedom to feel whatever you are feeling.

■ A CONSCIOUS LIVING PRACTICE FOR TODAY ■

Shift this moment to a more generous way of listening to yourself. Let go of your stance of critical listening. Give yourself an openhearted, open-minded acceptance for everything you're thinking and feeling. As you go through the world today, be aware of shifting into critical mode. When you notice you've started being hard on yourself, shift back into an easeful way of listening to yourself.

APRIL 24

We must love one another or die.——W. H. AUDEN

IN RELATIONSHIP

Let's take a moment to sum up what you think constitutes relationship. I no longer use the term *good relationship* because, in my belief, either you are *in relationship* or you are not. If it's not relationship, remember, it's entanglement.

- Both people are totally committed to employing the relationship as the arena for self-knowledge.
- Both people are committed to being close.
- Both people are committed to their own individual development.
- Both people tell all the truth, all the time. Anything else is an entanglement. No exceptions.
- Both people take full responsibility for themselves. There are no victims and no villains.
- Conflicts are resolved in a win/win manner. No one has to lose in order for someone else to win.
- Both people consistently demonstrate that they choose having a good time over being right and making the other person wrong.

■ A CONSCIOUS LIVING PRACTICE FOR TODAY ■

Say the following affirmation to yourself several times, taking the time to breathe deeply and slowly, and taking the time to feel the commitment deep in your body: I commit myself to the above ways of being in a relationship. I am willing to accept no less from myself or from my partner. I am willing to do whatever it takes to remove the obstacles I place in my own path and to clear a way toward conscious relationship.

That man is richest whose pleasures are the cheapest.—HENRY DAVID THOREAU

GOOD TIMES

Did I end my list yesterday with "I choose to have a good time over being right and making the other person wrong"? A good *time*? How can that be, when relationship is about struggle, about hard work, about slogging through the murky darkness of your soul in tandem with another?! Laura writes: I recently attended a wedding where the bride and groom had written their own vows, and as both are creative, loving people, I looked forward to hearing their words of affirmation and commitment. Instead, I heard a vow that sounded something like this: "We commit to doing the hard, painful work that is necessary to maintain a marriage in these troubled times. We promise to stand by each other during dark times and to support each other when it seems that the world or our marriage no longer does." The vows went on for quite a while in that vein. I listened, terribly saddened by their words. It is true that commitment involves riding out the waves, but where was the fun? What happened to joy? Their vows left out the promise to laugh together, to look lightly on the world and each other, to take the long, soul-filling walks that they so loved to take together. Relationship is *not* about misery or shouldering a cross; it is about joyfully walking together, recognizing that sometimes the path may be dark, but looking for and allowing yourself to feel the lightness in every step.

■ A CONSCIOUS LIVING PRACTICE FOR TODAY ■

Using the ten-second rule (anything that truly carries the essence of you and your feelings can be said in ten seconds or less), think about how you might phrase a vow for your own relationship. You will have to trim out a lot in order to keep it to ten seconds, but consider it good practice for reaching the core of who you are and what you want and need in a relationship.

....

If a man will begin with certainties, he shall end in doubts; but if he will be content to begin with doubts, he shall end in certainties.—FRANCIS BACON

BAROMETERS OF RELATIONSHIP HEALTH

At the core of the troubles that exist intrapersonally (within yourself) and interpersonally (in your relationship with others) lie three areas I have already discussed as methods for creating a relationship. These three methods—accepting feelings, telling the truth, and keeping your agreements—can also serve as a barometer for what and how much is wrong in a relationship. I urge you to ask the following questions as you begin to explore your relationships and chart a course toward conscious living within them:

• What truth is not being spoken here?
• What feelings are not being experienced or accepted here?
• What agreements have been broken here?

Try looking first within yourself to find answers to these questions.

■ A CONSCIOUS LIVING PRACTICE FOR TODAY ■

Today, give yourself time and space to ask and begin to know the answers to these wonderings:

A truth that I have difficulty knowing about myself is _____.
A feeling that is difficult for me to experience and to accept in
    myself is _____.
An agreement that I have broken with myself is _____.

Of all feats of skill, the most difficult is that of being honest.——MARIE DE BEAUSACQ

KNOWING FEELINGS

The ability to know your feelings deeply is more important than many of you realize. Many of you have spent a lifetime learning to hide your feelings. You may have even survived an early hostile environment partly by your ability to conceal your feelings. In conscious living, though, you realize that the act of hiding your feelings is what causes many communication breakdowns. Carried further, many doctors point out that the act of hiding your feelings from others is responsible for many emotional and physical ills. There is a high art to acknowledging your feelings deeply while learning to act on them effectively. The ability to know your feelings makes effective communication much more likely.

■ A CONSCIOUS LIVING PRACTICE FOR TODAY ■

Take five or ten minutes to remember yourself playing the childhood game of hide-and-seek. Where were you most likely to hide: in a closet or other small space, or in the open, such as behind a sofa? How did you feel as you heard the seeker's footsteps approaching, coming close to finding you? Did your heart pound? Did your breathing quicken? How are those feelings similar to ones you might have now when you are facing detection after you have hidden a thought, a feeling, a truth? Is there another way for you, a way that involves stepping out into the light?

APRIL 28

Always the beautiful answer who asks a more beautiful question.—E. E. CUMMINGS

ASKING HIGH-QUALITY QUESTIONS

The power of questions is immense, yet few of you really take advantage of that power in your daily conscious living. Many of you ask questions that are not really questions—they are really attacks in disguise or attempts to change another person: "Are you going to sit and watch television all day?" "Do you really need another pair of expensive shoes?" Today, make your questions count. Ask the highest-quality questions you can think up. Don't waste the power of questions on things you already know the answer to.

■ A CONSCIOUS LIVING PRACTICE FOR TODAY ■

Today, ask only questions to which you really, with all your heart, want answers. Pause for a moment right now and ask yourself: What are the most important questions I need to ask in order to make the most of my journey of conscious living?

....

APRIL 29

Life has got to be lived—that's all there is to it.—ELEANOR ROOSEVELT

THE BIG PICTURE

Keep the following big picture in the back of your mind: Get out your calculator and do a little math. Multiply your age times 365. If you want to be precise, add the number of days since your birthday. That will give you the number of days you've been breathing the air of this planet. Now subtract that number from 25,000, an average number of days an American lives. You might beat the average a little with good genes and healthy living, but, on the other hand, you might get on the wrong side of a bus next week. Once you get clear that you have x more times to wake up, it inspires you to do a more serious level of prioritizing. It inspires you to wonder: What's important?

■ A CONSCIOUS LIVING PRACTICE FOR TODAY ■

If you have done your math and figured out the number of days you have left, take a moment to ask yourself: What's important? Think through your day with that question in your mind. If this were your last day, would this be what you would want to do?

....

APRIL 30

Yet there isn't a train I wouldn't take no matter where it's going.
—EDNA ST. VINCENT MILLAY

A MAGICAL JOURNEY

Have you ever taken a trip that felt magical? Perhaps you went somewhere unfamiliar, to a place where the language, the food, and the customs felt foreign and exciting and magical. Or perhaps you returned to a place from your past and were able to relive moments of your life that hold fond, warm memories.

Laura writes: In my early thirties, with three young children, a full-time job, writing classes, and a volunteer position that took up a lot of time, I took a vacation—by myself. It was a gift to myself at a time when I needed quiet with near-desperation. For five days, I stayed in a hotel, and here's what I did: I ate when I wanted to eat. I slept when I was tired. I went swimming every day, and I wrote for hours, at whatever hours appealed to me. I visited with a dear friend and spent time laughing and feeling like someone I hadn't seen in a while—a younger, better-rested, lighter-hearted version of myself. At the end of the trip, I was delighted to return home to my children; I went back as a mother who was more present because I had taken the time to journey with myself. Those days are still magical to me, and I recall them when I am feeling pressured, overwhelmed, undervalued.

■ A CONSCIOUS LIVING PRACTICE FOR TODAY ■

Whether your life will allow you to take a trip as extended as the one Laura writes about, or whether you can only get away for a few hours, your work (and play!) today is to plan a "vacation" for yourself. Even an afternoon can be a vacation, but here are the rules:

- You get to choose where you're going.
- You get to choose how to spend the time.
- Your time must be spent on you and you alone.
- Your vacation is intended to be pure pleasure . . . plan it that way!

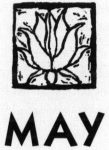

MAY

MAY 1

A lie would have no sense unless the truth were felt to be dangerous.—ALFRED ADLER

TRUTH-TELLING

For the next several days, I am going to spend time delving into truth-telling, talking about it and practicing it. Many of you spent so many years being separated from your truth that the journey back toward it can feel long and discouraging. You will discover, though, that your essence has a built-in reward system; as you journey toward truth, you will feel a lightness and joy that is the sound of your essence finding its voice and blossoming forth after too many years pushed into silence and hiding.

■ A CONSCIOUS LIVING PRACTICE FOR TODAY ■

As a prelude to telling the truth in relationship to others, practice knowing and telling the truth to yourself. Stand in front of a mirror at a time when you won't be interrupted, so you can abandon self-consciousness (which is simply an obstacle you allow yourself to set up) and breathe calmly and deeply, looking at yourself in the mirror. Tune in to your physical experience as you do so and make the following observations to yourself.

Right now I feel _____.
My head feels _____.
My shoulders feel _____.
I am most aware of my _____.
I'm aware of it because it feels _____.

You need to find out if this is a relationship in which you can experience both unity
with another person and the development of yourself as a separate being.
Can you be close and be yourself at the same time?

HONORING YOURSELF AND YOUR RELATIONSHIP

The central question for most people in a close relationship is: "Can I be me and still be with my partner?" You can learn the crucial skill of honoring your experience, who you are, and hearing your partner and honoring him or her. The ability to be present to your experience while in the company of another person, especially a romantic partner, is at the heart of building an enlightening relationship. What this requires is a commitment to knowing and honoring who you are; if you don't do this, you are at the whim of any strong fluctuations of mood and energy around you.

■ A CONSCIOUS LIVING PRACTICE FOR TODAY ■

Spend a few moments thinking about how you allow externals (events, or the way other people feel) to tell you how you should feel. Answer these questions in your heart and give them room to teach you.

When my partner is in a bad mood, I often feel _____.
When things don't go my way, I'll find myself thinking about "if only's" _____.
To take me from a great mood to a lousy one, all my partner has to do is _____.

Between whom there is hearty truth, there is love.——HENRY DAVID THOREAU

TRUTH AND CONSEQUENCES

For many people, *all* fears create the same feeling: it's not that you're afraid of truth as a concept; it's that you don't want to deal with the fall-out when it happens. There are simple ways to eliminate defensiveness in a relationship, though. Replacing it with wonder, for instance, is using a nondefensive communication pattern. If you truly accept and know your feelings and tell the truth, these patterns will flow naturally outward from that acceptance because you will be focused on your wonder rather than on your doubt or blame. Your intention to own what you feel is not yet internalized and true if your statements sound like this: "You made me angry." Instead, your statements will all begin with the "I" rather than with the "Thou," as Martin Buber, a well-known psychologist, postulates. Only you can know your truth, and only you are responsible for your truth. A key phrase that you will use on your journey toward owning your feelings will begin with "I feel," rather than with "You make me feel."

■ A CONSCIOUS LIVING PRACTICE FOR TODAY ■

Take a few moments alone and practice replacing the "you" statements with the "I" statements, saying them out loud. Notice the difference in the sound of your words when you replace the personal pronoun *you* with *I.*

You made me really angry.	I feel really angry.
You're irritating me again.	I feel irritated again.
You wouldn't want to go on a date, would you?	I'd like to go out with you.
You're confusing me.	I feel confused.

You're obviously upset about something.	I sense that you're upset.
You are frightening me right now.	I feel scared right now.

....

MAY 4

The man who speaks the truth is always at ease.——PERSIAN PROVERB

TELLING THE TRUTH ABOUT YOUR ANGER

When anger begins in your body, it often starts out feeling like a heady stimulant, making the heart and pulse race, giving you energy and perhaps even freeing you, allowing you to say things you would not normally say, to feel the hugeness of your emotions without apology. A person in early, clean anger can bring to mind the image of a hungry infant, consumed by rage without self-judgment. Even the infant, though, soon learns that rage rarely wins a positive response, and as adults, most of you have developed elaborate methods for subduing or denying or lying about your anger in order to avoid your own judgments and the judgments of others who see anger as messy and chaotic and frightening. The catch, of course, is that the more anger you subdue, the more anger you feel. I think of the scene early in *Fantasia*, where each time a bucket of water begins to empty out the floodwaters, ten more buckets appear and fill up the flooding castle. Without accepting your own anger, telling the truth about it, and making (and, of course, keeping) an agreement with yourself to find effective ways to handle your anger, you are not owning it and you will be unable to truly be in a conscious state within your own heart, much less in conscious relationship with another.

What one life experience might you choose to begin with in embracing your imperfection and the imperfections of those around you at the time?

Sometimes it is difficult to accept that it is your own resistance, rather than other people or the world, that is responsible for your problems.

....

MAY 5

What we think, that we become.——GANDHI

WHAT MATTERS MOST

In conscious living, one of the daily tasks is to focus your attention on what matters most. In the first session of counseling with people, I often ask them, "What matters to you most in the world?" Frequently their eyebrows shoot up in surprise, and many say it's the first time anyone's asked them that question. That's odd, isn't it? How peculiar that we can go through a day on this planet—one of the precious 25,000 days we get (on average)—without pausing to wonder if we are focusing on what matters most.

■ A CONSCIOUS LIVING PRACTICE FOR TODAY ■

Pause now and ask yourself this question: What matters most to me in my life? Let your mind and body answer freely. You may not like the answer you get, but it's always better to give even the unpopular response a good listening.

MAY 6

Truth has no special time of its own. Its hour is now—always.
—ALBERT SCHWEITZER

THE RULES OF INTEGRITY

Simplified, the rules of integrity are:

Rule One: Don't deny your feelings but don't wallow in them, either. Find an effective, straightforward, and non-blameful way to communicate feelings. If you're scared or angry, say so—no big deal.

Rule Two: Tell the whole truth. Make yourself safe for people to tell the truth to.

Rule Three: Be selective in making commitments and scrupulous about keeping them. Don't break commitments unless no other alternatives exist, and then carefully communicate about the broken commitment to all relevant people.

Rule Four: Take responsibility for any enterprise in which you're involved, and ask for each participant to do the same.

■ A CONSCIOUS LIVING PRACTICE FOR TODAY ■

Make a copy of these rules and post them in a conspicuous place so your friends, coworkers, and family can see them. If anyone asks about them, explain them and what they mean in your life. Even if no one asks about them, you will have a friendly reminder for yourself.

....

MAY 7

Dignity does not consist in possessing honours, but in deserving them.—ARISTOTLE

LOOKING INSIDE INTEGRITY BREAKDOWNS

In my role as therapist and consultant, I have had the opportunity to look inside the wreckage of many relationship disasters. What I often find are breakdowns of integrity. Usually the problem can be traced to a moment when someone did not tell the truth or keep a specific agreement. Many people tell me that they withheld the truth because they felt that telling the truth would break a sense of trust they enjoyed. What they do not realize is that the act of withholding the truth is what breaks the trust. Withholding destroys trust, and to get the trust back again usually requires the courageous act of acknowledging the withheld truth or broken agreement. This path is definitely "the road less traveled."

■ A CONSCIOUS LIVING PRACTICE FOR TODAY ■

Make it a top-priority goal today to communicate a withheld truth. First, make a commitment to doing it in a safe and effective way. Then, think of an appreciation you haven't told someone, or perhaps a regret or resentment. Make a point of telling the relevant person today, preferably via oral communication.

....

MAY 8

As if we could kill time without injuring eternity!—HENRY DAVID THOREAU

CLARIFYING YOUR PURPOSE

Purpose and intention are short, to-the-point statements of what you're up to in your life. There are big purposes and intentions, such as your purpose for your life and your intentions for your career, and there are more modest ones, such as your purpose for a given conversation. Whether you're dealing with a big or little purpose, there is a palpable shift in energy when you know your purpose.

Whenever I feel confused or out of sorts, I've trained myself to take a moment to review my purpose. Life is about drifting from your purpose, then catching the drift and getting back on track. It all hinges on knowing what your purpose is. I sat down one day in the seventies and spent an hour figuring out the purpose of my life. It may have been the most important hour of my whole existence. I express my chosen purpose like this: I grow in love and creativity every day, as I inspire others who are interested to do the same. In my seminars and workshops, I've invited thousands of people to sit down for an hour and clarify the purpose of their lives. Not one of them has ever said it was wasted time.

■ A CONSCIOUS LIVING PRACTICE FOR TODAY ■

Pause for ten seconds and select a grand purpose for your day—to grow, for example, in love and wisdom through every interaction. Think for a moment about a satisfying goal for your day. When you've selected one, picture it rolling out ahead of you throughout the day, as a splendid purple carpet might roll out ahead of your every step. Picture your purpose smoothing the way for your every interaction throughout this day of conscious living.

MAY 9

Keep me away from the wisdom which does not cry,
the philosophy which does not laugh . . . —KAHLIL GIBRAN

WINKS FROM THE UNIVERSE

Laura writes: A package arrives for me in the mail on a day when I am feeling particularly harried. I have spent the morning Christmas shopping amongst the other harried shoppers, and although I want to sit with a cup of coffee and a good book, I don't allow myself the respite. Despite loving writing and counting it among the several things I do in which I can lose myself totally and joyfully, I am viewing it as a chore as I start leafing through a stack of index cards in the package, research materials that are part of a writing project. One of the fifty or sixty cards falls onto the floor and I bend to pick it up. *It's been lovely, but I have to scream now,* it reads. That's all it says. I let the card stay on the floor and I collapse beside it in laughter. Immediately, I call to mind a phrase of Gay and Katie's: "a wink from the universe." In this case, it means permission to know the joy of the day, to give myself a gift, to let go of the seriousness of it all for at least a while. I spend the rest of the afternoon sipping good coffee and losing myself in a wonderful novel, and when evening comes, I feel restored and focused and able to attend to my work again, but, miraculously, it no longer carries the weight of work.

■ A CONSCIOUS LIVING PRACTICE FOR TODAY ■

Identify one thing that you have wanted to do over the last several weeks but haven't done because it seems too self-indulgent, because your life seems too busy, because you don't feel like you deserve whatever it is. Give yourself permission to do it, and keep the agreement with yourself.

The thing I have wanted to do is to _____.
I am going to do this on (date) _____.

MAY 10

I seem to have been like a child playing on the seashore, finding now and then a prettier shell than ordinary, whilst the great ocean of truth lay undiscovered before me.
—ISAAC NEWTON

PRIORITIZING

Prioritizing is a key skill in conscious living. Through correct prioritizing, visions become reality. In Anne Lamott's excellent book on creativity, *Bird by Bird,* she recalls her father's wise advice to her brother. He had put off a term paper on birds of America until the night before it was due, and he was fretting and stewing at the kitchen table, surrounded by books, encyclopedias, and paraphernalia. The father put an arm around the boy and said, "Bird by bird, buddy. Just take it bird by bird." This is always how great visions get implemented—one step at a time.

Prioritizing, fortunately, is a skill that can be learned. It is wonderful if you are blessed with an organic gift for it, but few are. I am not so blessed. I just use prosaic old "to do" lists, crossing off and adding on items, one foot in front of the other and bird by bird.

■ A CONSCIOUS LIVING PRACTICE FOR TODAY ■

Do a one-minute experiment in prioritizing. Jot down the top-five things you want to accomplish today. Now, put a 1 by the one you most dread doing, a 2 by the one you dread doing a little less, and so on. As an experiment, today do the one you most dread doing first. The rest of your day may feel like vacation.

....

MAY 11

When we are afraid, everything rustles.—SOPHOCLES

THE FOUR FACES OF FEAR

When we're afraid, we express it in four major ways: Fight, Freeze, Flee, and Faint. In my workshops I call these the Four F's. Some people get angry and lash out when they're scared. They're the Fighters, and it's important to know that it's fear that drives their anger. Other people get immobile and tongue-tied when they're scared; they're the Freezers. A third group gets spacey and confused; they're the Fainters. Finally, some people run, withdraw, pull back, and hide when they get scared; they're the Flee-ers.

In counseling people for the past thirty years, I've found that the majority of people are Fighters and Flee-ers, with Freezers and Fainters in the minority. I've seen many people's lives changed by learning which response to fear they have. For example, knowing that when you're angry you're also scared can be a major learning for people who get angry a lot. When people can learn to say "I'm scared" rather than ranting about their anger, they often soften in front of my eyes.

■ A CONSCIOUS LIVING PRACTICE FOR TODAY ■

As you move through your day, look for your different responses to fear. Find out if you're a Fighter, a Flee-er, a Freezer, or a Fainter. When you can identify your major way of responding to fear, begin to train yourself to acknowledge your fear to yourself and others.

....

MAY 12

The biggest disease today is not leprosy or tuberculosis, but rather the feeling of being unwanted.—MOTHER TERESA OF CALCUTTA

DIGESTING YOURSELF

When you swallow your feelings, your body begins to digest itself. Ulcers, heart disease, cancer—all have been shown to have a relationship with stress. While stress may or may not create bacteria and cause renegade genes to mutate, it undeniably creates an environment that is welcoming and supportive of physiological processes that can—that *will*—ultimately kill you. If you visualize the process, you can see what repression does to the lightness and magic of the human body; imagine the sharpness of your strongest feelings, whether feelings of joy or anger or sadness. When strong, sharp feelings are hidden deep inside like shameful secrets, the feelings tear at your organs and block the path that your blood wants to travel as it gives you life. Expression keeps you open and strong, able and ready to easily defend your physical health and emotional well-being. Instead of concentrating on fighting or fleeing or otherwise denying feelings, your body is doing what it was intended for all along: living in a state of peaceful acceptance and essence.

■ A CONSCIOUS LIVING PRACTICE FOR TODAY ■

Read through the following paragraph, finishing the sentences in your thoughts:

The feeling that I most often hide inside of me is _____. I hide this feeling because it seems _____ to me. When I hide or repress it, I can feel the sensation in my _____. It feels _____. I know that repressing this feeling is not good for me physically or emotionally, and I know that repressing this feeling keeps me from being totally inside of relationship. I commit to letting this feeling live its full expression and I commit to honoring, accepting, and telling the truth about this feeling.

You perpetrate dis-ease on yourself every time you create a gap between how you actually are and how you pretend to be.

....

MAY 13

We take our shape, it is true, within and against that cage of reality bequeathed to us at our birth, and yet it is precisely through our dependence on this reality that we are most endlessly betrayed.—JAMES BALDWIN

ZEN COMFORT

Sometimes a dose of reality, administered with love and good timing, can be the best medicine of all. A Zen student told me the following story, allegedly true: A Zen master telephoned one of his students, a woman who was dying of cancer. Friends, gathered around her, were surprised to hear her laugh at something he said. When she got off the phone she looked cheerful for the first time in days. The wisdom he imparted turned out to be nothing like they expected. He had told her,

"Don't even think for a moment that you're not going to die!" On the surface this might not sound like a comforting thing to say to a dying person; on such occasions people often like to paint a pretty picture of The Great Beyond. But the Zen master knew in his heart that reality—this moment!—has all the spiritual liberation in it that anyone really needs, and his student knew it in her heart, too.

■ A CONSCIOUS LIVING PRACTICE FOR TODAY ■

Look at your face in the mirror. Imagine for a moment that the face looking back at you is the face of a Zen master. Tell yourself something as important and real as the Zen master in the story above told his student. What is it that the Zen master in you most needs to say to you?

....

MAY 14

Most of the shadows of this life are caused by our standing in our own sunshine.
—RALPH WALDO EMERSON

COUNT YOUR BLESSINGS

Just above the desk where Laura writes is a cross-stitch that says "Count Your Blessings." Stuck in the corners are pictures of her three young boys. When life gets most chaotic and difficult, the ironies of the pictures and the cross-stitch are a source of amusement and a reminder that there will always be dissonance in our lives—the very things that bring you the most joy are also the things that can bring you the most confusion and anguish. Kahlil Gibran wrote of grief in this same light. He said that your grief is proportionate to the joy you have known with another in relationship; the more you love, the more you feel loss when that love is changed. It is only natural that the depth of your pain corresponds to the depth of your love. I believe in reframing your confusion and pain and seeing it as an invitation to learning and to wondering. In your times of greatest distress, you are being given the gift of choice: shall you take the path you have traveled many times before, furthering your anguish, or shall you learn, wonder, grow, change, take a new path? The choice is yours.

■ A CONSCIOUS LIVING PRACTICE FOR TODAY ■

Find time for yourself—five minutes, ten—and sit somewhere quiet. Read through the sentence below, answering the question to yourself. When the question is answered, take your five or ten minutes to simply sit with the feelings that were generated about your greatest present pain. Beware of the part of you that will want to solve and absolve. Simply be with the pain.

Right now in my life, the greatest pain that I feel is because of _____.

I commit to knowing about this pain and I commit to learning where it came from and where it might lead me that I haven't been before.

....

MAY 15

Humankind cannot bear very much reality.—T. S. ELIOT

THE COST OF SETTLING

Not long ago at the library, I ran into a friend I hadn't seen for a couple of years. I was shocked inside when I saw him. His face was drawn and haggard, and he looked ten years older than the vibrant thirty-five-year-old I remembered from before. I expressed my concern and asked him what he'd been going through. He said he'd been having a lot of marital struggles, but that he'd eventually got them straightened out. Skeptical of his answer, I asked him how he'd solved his problems. What he said chilled my heart. He said he'd lowered his expectations and decided to settle for less than what he wanted. I shared my lack of enthusiasm for this solution, and pointed out that it looked like it was causing him stress. He backed away from me quickly and said, "That's my decision and I'm sticking to it." I felt deeply saddened by his choice, then I realized the reason I felt sad was that I was probably doing the same thing unconsciously in areas of my life.

■ A CONSCIOUS LIVING PRACTICE FOR TODAY ■

Pause to reflect on key areas of your life. Are you settling for less in any of those areas? Are there other ways you could approach those areas that wouldn't involve compromising your values and desires?

....

MAY 16

Could a greater miracle take place than for us to look through each other's eyes for an instant?—HENRY DAVID THOREAU

MIRACLES MADE OF MAGIC

A miracle is made of magic. It is, by its very definition, something that most people believe wasn't supposed to happen—that is, of course, what makes it a miracle. A child is born to an infertile couple; a terminally ill person lives long past the early estimates; two people are somewhere they never intended to be and meet and fall in love; each of these occurrences might be called a miracle. Some miracles, then, are winks from the universe—huge and life changing and fate charged. Others, though, are waiting to happen in each choice you make, in each moment of your life. While you are waiting for fate to play its hand, a thousand miracle moments might pass you by. Take control! Know that you are in charge of the chance to have miracles in your life, your love, your relationship.

■ A CONSCIOUS LIVING PRACTICE FOR TODAY ■

Spend a few moments today thinking about, celebrating, and creating intentions for these things:

A miracle that has occurred in my life.
What part I played in making that miracle.
A miracle that I want in my life.
The part I will play in making it happen.

The moment you stop pretending, your healing begins.

....

MAY 17
Life is a voyage that's homeward bound.—HERMAN MELVILLE

LIMITING SELF-ESTEEM

The fear of outdoing someone else—and ultimately of leaving others behind—is deeply rooted in your mind and body. Therapists in Australia call this the "tall poppy syndrome." The goal is not to stand out too tall above the other poppies blossoming in the fields. Many particularly gifted people hold themselves back from reaching their full potential because to do so would mean outshining someone else—and the someone, I should note, is often located in the distant past. You fear the loss and loneliness of abandoning others, even those who are distant ghosts.

■ A CONSCIOUS LIVING PRACTICE FOR TODAY ■

Think about a way in which you may have held yourself back from success for fear of outshining someone else. Are you still doing so today?

- Who are you trying to protect?
- How are you damaging yourself?
- How can you let go of the chains you put around yourself?

MAY 18

Now faith is the substance of things hoped for,
the evidence of things not seen.—HEBREWS 11:1

SOUL CHOICES

For the next several weeks, your journey will take you through a set of soul choices that I believe are essential for relationship to flourish. Within these soul choices, I include six co-commitments, which you may recognize if you have read *Conscious Loving* or *The Conscious Heart*. The co-commitments provide a solid, safe foundation for change; they also expose the counter-commitments, which are barriers that aren't apparent prior to entering into a relationship. As you begin to read and think about the soul choices, listen to your heart; let the sounds of fear or anxiety mingle with the sounds of hope and excitement like guests gathering in the home of your body. Honor the many conflicting voices you may hear—let them be heard, accept them, and embrace them so that you can continue to move forward on your journey.

■ A CONSCIOUS LIVING PRACTICE FOR TODAY ■

- Today I commit to continuing on my path of wonder.
- Today I commit to welcoming and embracing and honoring all of my feelings.
- Today I commit to giving special attention to the feelings that make me most uncomfortable, letting them rest comfortably or uncomfortably in my body and embracing those feelings, doing nothing to chase them away.

You get in the habit of protecting yourself at an early age by pretending not to be the way you are.

Life shrinks or expands in proportion to one's courage.——Anaïs Nin

COMMITTING TO COMMITMENT

Commitment: *I commit to being close and I commit to clearing up anything in the way of doing so.*

Counter-Commitment: *I commit to holding back and to keeping hidden my barriers to closeness.*

In the film *As Good as It Gets,* Jack Nicholson plays a middle-aged man who suffers from obsessive-compulsive disorder. His mental illness rules his life, and he turns bitter and nasty because of his lack of connection with others. When he falls in love and is unable to maintain a relationship because of his symptoms, he finally addresses his illness and works toward clearing up the things that stand in the way of full closeness with another. He makes the decision to do so after looking at his life and his loneliness and asking in despair, "What if this is as good as it gets?" If the choice is to hold back, to "protect" oneself, loneliness and despair *is* as good as it gets. If you make the choice of committing to full closeness, the possibilities are endless.

■ A CONSCIOUS LIVING PRACTICE FOR TODAY ■

Wonder—do not judge, do not doubt—about yourself today:

A reason that I put up barriers to closeness: _____.
A way in which I put up barriers to closeness: _____.

Affirmation: *I commit myself to full closeness and to clearing up anything within me that stands in the way.*

*A person will be called to account on Judgment Day for everything
permissible he could have enjoyed and did not.*—TALMUD

COMMITMENT AND COUNTER-COMMITMENT

Contrast these two statements:

I commit to my own complete development as an individual.

I commit to holding back from expressing my full development as
an individual.

Most of us are in a tug-of-war between these two commitments. If
the first one wins, we get to be happy and fulfilled to the core. If the second one wins, we know it deep in our core and, usually, so does everyone else.

Nowhere is individual development more important than in an intimate relationship. Even if two people are deeply committed to union
with each other, their commitment to development as solo entities con-
tributes as much to the health of the relationship as their focus on
union. A couple volunteered for a demonstration during a relationship
workshop Kathlyn and I were teaching. They expressed a desire to
develop as individuals—they felt they were too dependent on each
other. Just to have an ice-breaking starting point, I asked them what
some of their favorite activities were. Without a moment's hesitation,
she said, "He loves golf." He replied, "She loves to cook." The audience
laughed, noticing that they had answered for each other rather than
expressing their own individual likes. Hearing the laughter, the couple
looked puzzled. "What's the joke?"

They clearly had a lot of work to do.

Say each of the commitments above two or three times out loud, getting a sense of how they feel in your body and mind.

Occasionally today, circulate the following affirmation through your mind: *I commit to my full development as an individual.*

....

MAY 21

Him that I love, I wish to be free—even from me.—ANNE MORROW LINDBERGH

EMPOWERING OTHERS

Commitment: *I commit to the full empowerment of people around me.*

Counter-Commitment: *I commit to holding back those around me so that they won't leave, so they'll need me, because I'm comfortable.*

At the core of the commitment to full empowerment is the power struggle that occurs between the twin needs for unity and autonomy I discussed on March 22. From your earliest moments of life, your soul simultaneously yearns for connection with others and struggles to maintain autonomy within connection. A commitment to full empowerment for the others in your life is necessarily based on your own sense of safety in autonomy. If you tailor your behavior to attempt to keep others from leaving you and to make yourself indispensable, you will hold them back in one way or another. The only way to empower others fully is to become fully empowered yourself, to let go of your fears of autonomy. The magic of this is that you will discover, once you have done so, that you are less alone, more unified, because your connections will be real relationship rather than dependent, fear-driven entanglement.

To empower, first you must release those parts of yourself that hold you hostage. Today, spend a few moments thinking and feeling the answers to the sentences that follow.

I am most frightened of being left by _____.
I will let go of my fear and honor my commitment to full empowerment by _____.

Affirmation: *I commit to the full empowerment of people around me.*

....

MAY 22

If we can change our thoughts, we can change the world.—H. M. TOMLINSON

HEALTHY RESPONSIBILITY

Again today, contrast two commitments:

I commit to taking full, healthy responsibility in my close relationships.
I commit to a lifelong search to find who's to blame for the fix I'm in.

Let me share a passage a man sent me after reading about responsibility in one of my books:

Up until I was around thirty, I don't think I ever took responsibility for what went on in my relationships. When the pressure was on, I always blamed the other person. Then I had a wake-up call: I realized that the same things kept happening, even if the relationship partners changed! It became very hard to blame it on the other person (though it didn't stop me from trying from time to time). My big issue was loneliness, so when I got in a relationship and felt lonely, I would blame it on the other person never being there for me. The problem was, I sought out people who would assume that they were at fault. I learned that for every person who wants to avoid responsibility, there's another person out there who's willing to take it for them.

■ A CONSCIOUS LIVING PRACTICE FOR TODAY ■

Take a look around your life: Your health, your love life, your job history. Describe these areas, taking full responsibility for them. Use sentences like these: "I do asthma now and then" (rather than "I have asthma"), "I arranged to get fired from my last job," "I create the feeling of depression in my body and mind sometimes."

....

MAY 23

Were we fully to understand the reasons for other people's behavior, it would all make sense.—SIGMUND FREUD

OPENING UP

Commitment: *I commit to revealing rather than concealing.*
Counter-Commitment: *I commit to hiding.*
Having another truly know you—at your deepest core—is at once one of the most fearful and intoxicating of human experiences. The fear stems from the worry that if you are truly known, you will not be loved, and the intoxication stems from the heady exhilaration of being able to let down your guard and be seen as you truly are. It is a paradox that unity, the very need that drives you toward relationship, is also the need that encourages you to make the choice to hide yourself. We desperately long for unity, for full connection with another, and are so fearful of rejection that we keep ourselves distant, hidden, safe. Until you make the

commitment to revealing, to letting another know you as you truly are, you will not know true relationship. Your personas may become entangled with another's, but you, your essence, will not live in relationship.

■ A CONSCIOUS LIVING PRACTICE FOR TODAY ■

When you find that you are most frightened in relationship, allow yourself to step back and to use breathing to get in touch with your essence, the parts of your essence that fear being known. Breathe deeply, inhaling and exhaling, as you let yourself feel and know your fear, and then continue breathing to carry you through a miracle move, as you tell another the truth of yourself: I feel frightened of being known. See where it takes you, honesty.

Affirmation: *I commit to revealing rather than concealing.*

....

MAY 24

Man is as full of potentiality as he is of impotence.——GEORGE SANTAYANA

COMMITTING TO JOY

Commitment: *I commit to having a good time in my close relationships.*

Counter-Commitment: *I commit to suffering, to finding out how much pain I can endure without flinching.*

It is an old stereotype, the John Wayne stoic who takes a bullet in the gut with a grunt, if that, but keeps on going, suffering in silence. Our culture tends to reward the stoic, the "Emotional Energizer Bunny" who keeps going and going and going. I encourage a more accepting approach to the forthright expression of emotional truth, no matter how messy that truth may be. The same is true for joy: is there any part of our culture that is truly comfortable with the gleeful, exuberant expression of joy and fun and laughter? From your earliest days, you are pressured into reining in the laughter in your heart: *Settle down! Indoor voices! That's not funny!* You hear these messages and many more that tell you that it is not all right to enjoy the ride. Life, love, and work are supposed to be suffered, not enjoyed—or so goes conventional American wisdom. It is time to let go of the judging voices and to let yourself feel the joy and humor that was silenced within you but wants to break free.

■ A CONSCIOUS LIVING PRACTICE FOR TODAY ■

Let yourself see the world differently today. In each instance when you feel frustrated (traffic is slow; you drop something; work doesn't go as you wished), let yourself find the humor in the situation. Sit back, breathe deeply, and feel laughter in your belly replace tightness and tension.

Affirmation: *I commit to having a good time in my close relationships.*

....

MAY 25

The young man knows the rules, but the old man knows the exceptions.
—OLIVER WENDELL HOLMES

ON THE CARPET

Laura writes: My newly-four-year-old son knocks over a glass of grape juice on the off-white carpet. It is the permanent kind of deep purple juice, the type that will tell mothers and fathers a hundred years from now that once small children lived here. *Thank you,* I say, sighing, meaning everything *but* thank you. I sink to the floor to begin repairing the damage. Looking up I see Timothy touching his forehead as if he is removing a top hat; with a melodramatic, sweeping gesture, he bows nearly to the floor as he says, "It is my *greatest* pleasure." It is my moment of choice, is it not? Later, I relive that moment: the frustration, the anger, the exhaustion of one more spill, one more chore, one more damn thing to do . . . but what stays with me all these months later is his voice accepting my thanks, his Sir Laurence Olivier performance, and my sudden break with irritation as I went gratefully sliding into laughter. We spent five minutes dissolved in giggles in each other's arms on the floor . . . and the grape juice? It waited. It can always wait; a four-year-old is four for only so long. And now, whenever I pass the fading purple stain, what I see is not the color of frustration or exhaustion; what I see is a moment when my young son and I lay on the floor together laughing, touching, sharing a moment of closeness. So much of life is like that: choices between anger and letting go of anger, holding tight to resentment like it will warm you or allowing yourself to be stripped bare until you can see the humanity and the humor in yourself and others.

■ A CONSCIOUS LIVING PRACTICE FOR TODAY ■

Today you will reframe something that happens. When you reframe, you choose to view something through a new or different lens (it is the old "half empty or half full" concept at work). The event itself hasn't changed; your *interpretation* is what changes. In the grape juice example, Laura chose to reframe; instead of seeing it as an opportunity for anger, she reframed it into an opportunity for closeness.

The event: _____.
The old interpretation: _____.
The new interpretation: _____.

....

MAY 26

I am a part of all that I have met.—ALFRED LORD TENNYSON

INTENTIONS BEHIND SPEAKING AND LISTENING

Every word you speak has an intention behind and beneath it. If you say something simple like, "How are you?" to a friend, you may have the intention of actually learning something about the person's emotional depths. If you say, "How are you?" to a person you hardly know, you may only have the intention of being polite. You may not actually want to know how the person really is. It's the intention behind the word that's important. The same is true for listening. Every moment of listening has an intention behind it. In one case you may be listening with the intention of rebutting the other person. In another case you're listening to get the person to like you. The intention beneath your listening is the real issue—each person's listening is as different as a thumbprint.

■ A CONSCIOUS LIVING PRACTICE FOR TODAY ■

Today focus on being aware of the shifting intentions behind your speaking and listening. Notice, for example, when you're "listening to criticize" versus "listening to support." Notice when you're "speaking to open possibilities" versus "speaking to be right."

....

MAY 27

I will act as if I do make a difference.—WILLIAM JAMES

THE DANGEROUS TRUTH

The idea of telling the truth seems dangerous to many people, but it is actually only dangerous if you resist it. I have seen the truth of that statement firsthand many hundreds of times in the therapy office. Over and over couples who are sorting out a problem caused only by lying about something come into my office. And the number-one reason they give for lying? They didn't want to hurt the feelings of the other person. One memorable couple whom I counseled had failed to tell each other about more than twenty affairs during the course of their twelve years together. When I asked them why they'd engaged in this epic deception, they gave two reasons: We didn't want to hurt the other, and we didn't want to destroy the trust between us!

One of the big delusions of life is thinking we have control over how other people feel. If we fall for this delusion, we will try to hide the truth so that people will feel the way we want them to feel. In marriage, politics, and life in general, this move inevitably leads to disaster.

■ A CONSCIOUS LIVING PRACTICE FOR TODAY ■

As you go through your day, you will encounter dozens of opportunities to tell the truth or hide it. You'll also have opportunities to hear the truth or shield yourself from it.

Do some simple experiments in truth-telling. To a grocery clerk, for example, you might say, "I feel pressured when it's crowded like it is today. Do you ever feel that way?" Speak the truth simply, and leave room in the conversation for others to do so.

....

MAY 28

There is nothing noble about being superior to some other man. The nobility is in being superior to your previous self.—HINDU PROVERB

RESPONSIBILITY AND RELATIONSHIP

Where does responsibility fit into your priorities about relationship? It's a question that is worth asking daily—and sometimes minute by minute. There are so many levels to responsibility: the questions about daily chores and how you view the labor of life, the questions about acknowledging the ways in which you hurt others, and the questions about how you impact on the world around you. Try to reduce responsibility to its simplest level for a moment. Imagine that you return home, exhausted after a tough day of work, and see that someone has dropped a mountain of trash in front of your door. What do you do?

Do you enter through the back door of the house? Do you call the local government angrily and demand that something be done? Do you wade through the garbage, leaving it, or do you—with frustration, quite likely—gather plastic bags and begin cleaning up the mess, perhaps even adding it to a compost heap or recycling bins when you finish? There will be times when all manners of things, including garbage, will be dumped in your path. How you view that garbage (as compost material, for instance, ready to enrich the soil of your relationship), and what you do with that garbage are key elements in your general approach to relationship. The essential question about responsibility is like the Watergate riff: *What did I do, and when did I do it?* and, most important, *What can I now do to create the outcome I desire?*

■ A CONSCIOUS LIVING PRACTICE FOR TODAY ■

For the next twenty-four hours, "Watergate" your approach to the tasks that surround you. Each time you face a task, whether it is one you enjoy or detest, ask yourself:

- How (if at all) did I create this task that is facing me?
- What actions of mine have created what now faces me?
- What do I get out of this task?
- What can I now do to create the outcome I desire?

MAY 29

I am as bad as the worst, but, thank God,
I am as good as the best.—WALT WHITMAN

THE DEVIL MADE ME DO IT

Once, teaching an undergraduate class on interpersonal communication, I had a student who approached me after class saying, with great relief, that the "I" language I was teaching would help her immensely in her relationship. She had been arguing a lot with her boyfriend, and the arguing always turned mean, with name-calling and accusations. My simple suggestion that partners take responsibility for their feelings, saying, "I feel angry," rather than blaming and saying, "You made me feel angry" or, worse, "You are an idiot," seemed to bring great hope to this young woman. She promised to try this approach. A few days later, she angrily accused me of presenting a theory that doesn't work in real life. With a few questions, I reached the core of the situation. In an argument that had rapidly escalated, she remembered the lessons I taught—or so she believed. Proudly displaying her new communication skills, she announced to her partner, "I *feel* that you're a jerk!" Oddly enough, he still got defensive. Ever so gently, I explained to my young student that "I feel that you're a jerk" hardly meets the criteria for nondefensive, responsible communication. The secret, I have learned, is that if you put the word *that* after the words *I feel*, you're offtrack. A feeling is a feeling (anger, pride, joy); anything else is almost undoubtedly an accusation.

■ A CONSCIOUS LIVING PRACTICE FOR TODAY ■

Today, try converting your feelings from a "you" orientation to an "I" orientation. You're doing this because it creates a less defensive communication environment and because it helps you to take responsibility for what you create.

"You" Orientation: You made me late for work again!

"I" Orientation: I feel frustrated that I allowed myself to be talked into helping you when I knew I'd be late for work.

You can see that with the "I" orientation you are much more likely to take healthy responsibility for it.

*The days come and go like muffled and veiled figures sent from a distant friendly party,
but they say nothing, and if we do not use the gifts they bring, they carry
them silently away.*—RALPH WALDO EMERSON

THE COST OF CHANGE

What do you do if someone asks you to change? Do you weigh the
costs to yourself if the change occurs, and the costs to the other if it
doesn't? For many of you, your self is hard-won, a building you have created from the ground up, sometimes at considerable cost as you have
added on the bricks, the stones, the trim work of personality. Many of
you jealously guard the sanctity of your self as if, at any moment, the fire
of another's feeling might rip through the corridors and rooms, turning
them to ash. There is a time, however, for compromise, a time for allowing the walls and floors and ceilings of self to become soft, giving, open
to change. There is a time when you should allow others to enter your
life and, as the result of their footsteps on the hallowed ground of self,
leave a mark that makes you different and, somehow, better.

■ A CONSCIOUS LIVING PRACTICE FOR TODAY ■

Identify a part of yourself that is most like a condemned house. It's
unsafe. It doesn't work for the occupant. It provides a shaky foundation
at best. What are you going to do to either shore up the foundation or
rebuild?

Today, put your energy into thinking creatively about these two
things:

• The part to change.
• How you're going to change it.

Your request for no MSG was ignored.—MESSAGE IN FORTUNE COOKIE

ARE YOU HAVING THE RIGHT EXPERIENCE?

At every moment you have both the chance to resist the learning opportunity it brings—by pretending you are having the wrong experience—and the chance to embrace the learning opportunity by assuming you are having the correct experience. If you hit three red lights in a row some morning when you're in a hurry, you could miss the whole learning potential of the experience by indignantly claiming that you're having the wrong experience. Or you could grow in wisdom by wondering, "What does hitting three red lights have to teach me that I need to learn right now?" The moment you open to learning, you get the wisdom right now. If you keep resisting, you usually don't get the message until later.

A woman in one of my workshops provided a good example of this principle. She said that in one day she got a speeding ticket, ran out of gas during rush hour on the busiest street in San Francisco, and broke her toe crossing the street. To her great credit, though, she didn't do a "poor me" riff on the experience. Instead, she asked herself, "What's going on here?" Immediately she got an insight about her relationship with time. She needed to slow down, not try to be in two places at the same time.

■ A CONSCIOUS LIVING PRACTICE FOR TODAY ■

Begin your day with an affirmation: *Today I open to the learning opportunities in every moment.* Say the sentence a few times in your mind, then take a few deep breaths while you let it settle into your body. Carry it with you today—remind yourself of it now and then as you embrace the challenges of your life.

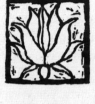

JUNE

JUNE 1

A lady of forty-seven who has been married twenty-seven years and has six children knows what love really is and once described it for me like this: Love is what you've been through with somebody.—JAMES THURBER

THE RELATIONSHIP DANCE

You choose partners who will bring your deepest hidden fears to the surface. Unfortunately, when those fears come to the surface, you often blame the other person for causing them. You don't realize that it was your own inspired choice of partners—driven by your need to grow beyond your fears—that brought the material to the surface. If you don't find your way out of this trap, you often pull back from the relationship and recycle the fears in some other relationship.

The conscious living (and loving) alternative: when your fears come up in relationships, take responsibility for them. Don't blame others for causing them. Instead, thank them for helping enlighten you, and ask for their support in helping you move through your fears to greater intimacy.

An example, if cliché: the commitment-phobic bachelor who has a twenty-year run, say, of shallow relationships and bemoans the lack of constancy and faithfulness in his love life. What might he discover if, when he first feels fear in a new relationship, he owns his fear? What if instead of blaming his new partner for wanting too much too fast he were to acknowledge that perhaps he is the one who feels tremendous need—and thus tremendous fear?

■ A CONSCIOUS LIVING PRACTICE FOR TODAY ■

Think of one or two people who bring up the deepest emotions in you. Who pushes your buttons? Reach out to those people today—with a talk or a call or a note—and thank them for bringing you such powerful learnings.

Life is hopeless but not serious.——HUNGARIAN PROVERB

THE LIFE-GAME

Comparing life to a game is an ancient metaphor. Based on a conversation I had with my daughter when she was seven, I discovered that children even make the comparison. Walking her to school, I often popped philosophical questions to her such as "Where do you think God is?" or "What's the most important thing in life?" There was never a shortage of answers. One day I asked, "What do you think life is?" Without missing a beat, she said, "A game." "And what's the purpose of the game?" I inquired. She thought for a moment, then said, "Having fun, and helping people if they fall down." What professor of philosophy could do better than that?

■ A CONSCIOUS LIVING PRACTICE FOR TODAY ■

Think of your life as a game. What role have you taken in the game? Are you playing passionately, for the sheer joy of it? Or have you decided to play halfheartedly or not at all?

As you move through your day, notice whether you are satisfied with the game you've created and the way you've chosen to play it.

JUNE 3

Be where you are; otherwise you will miss your life.—BUDDHA

THE CONSTANT SHIFT

One of the big insights of the Buddha was that nature, the universe, and we, its citizens, are all in a state of constant change. This insight has powerful practical value in daily life. If we know, for example, that the mood we're in will shift of its own accord, we're less likely to panic when we're in a bad one or overcharge our credit cards when we're in a good one. If we know that sadness or anger will soon melt into some other feeling, we're less likely to try to force those feelings to go away. If we relax and let go, they'll pass by themselves.

I learned this lesson vividly one evening while on a solo retreat in a remote mountain cabin. I began feeling lonely, so I tried to call a few friends. No one was home. Still feeling lonely, I busied myself with a card game. Soon I was feeling even more lonely, because I wanted someone to play with. After a while I realized that the more I tried to get rid of the loneliness, the more it gripped me. Rather than push it away, I began to investigate it. Where did I feel it in my body? Was it heaviness or pressure or tension? Within a few moments the feeling had dissolved completely, replaced by a sense of adventure and calm.

■ A CONSCIOUS LIVING PRACTICE FOR TODAY ■

Take a moment to think of yourself as a vast space with a lot of activity in it. For example, think of yourself as a rainforest or a big city. Get a sense of the millions of processes and activities taking place in the vastness of you. Everything is in flux; everything is on the move. Give all of those activities room to happen—let everything move and flow and change.

As you move (and flow and change) through your day, return occasionally to the sense of yourself as a vast space with immense movement in it.

JUNE 4

Blessed are they who heal us of self-despisings.
Of all services which can be done to man,
I know of none more precious.——WILLIAM HALE WHITE

AWAKENING

If you have ever had surgery, you may have a vague memory of the moments when you began to awaken from the anesthesia. From some deep, dark place, you began to surface. The surfacing is not always easy; the unconsciousness presses down upon you even as your conscious self tries to push upward and emerge. Once you reach a conscious state, you find yourself in some strange place that is both painful and giddy. So it is with the choice to live the emotionally and relationally conscious life. Having spent so many years blanketed by denial and defenses, the letting go and coming to life—to conscious life—is sometimes a struggle. Your heart may protest: *I am not strong enough! I can't bear the bright yellow light of reality; I will break from the strength of the honesty that surrounds me!* This is not true, of course, but having not yet come out on the other side of consciousness, how can you be sure of its safety? You *could* trust *my* word—it is trustworthy. Or you could trust the feelings that you experience as you begin this journey, the breakthrough feelings of excitement, of hope, the glow of the truth the first time you let yourself speak it. Loosen your hold on a half-lived life and jump fully into the rich, brilliant, blinding colors of consciousness. Having been bathed in the light of conscious loving and living, you will never choose to return to the old ways.

■ A CONSCIOUS LIVING PRACTICE FOR TODAY ■

How do you wake up in the morning? Are you easy to awaken? Difficult? Do you moan and groan and complain, or do you bounce out of bed with energy and enthusiasm? Think about the way you awaken, and you will learn something important about the way that you face life in general.

....

JUNE 5

No one can make you feel inferior without your consent.—ELEANOR ROOSEVELT

PASSIVITY-AGGRESSION

In these days of easy-access psychological theory, with books, movies, and even sitcoms throwing around terms that used to be reserved for the darkened offices and leather couches of the analysts, the phrase *passive-aggressive* gets plenty of airplay. In its fifteen minutes of Warholian fame, the phrase lost its power; people lightly accuse others of being passive-aggressive and perform armchair diagnoses on the most casual of acquaintances. Give passivity and aggression—and the marriage of the two—your attention for a few days, though. Explore the partners and their pairing, because more than many other defenses, passive-aggressive behavior is a standard shot at people moving toward a conscious life in direct opposition to those around them.

First, the threat: Why is your commitment to honesty, to agreement-keeping, to acceptance of yourself and others, so loaded for those around you? It is a question well worth asking. The answer that resonates most deeply is that when you move into a conscious stance, you sometimes reflect back to significant others a less than flattering portrait of their own lives. Where you are joy and lightness, the friend living a half-life is anger and weight. Where you are truth, the parent trapped in old, tired patterns is deception. Where you are a lightning rod for sparks of creativity and blazing fires of warmth, the lover is a tight, uncomfortable mass of chilled repression. You all serve as mirrors for others; through relationship, you see yourself in certain ways, but when you clean the mirror—although I believe that you will be delighted with the reflection that greets you—others, seeing their own reflection next to yours, may feel pale and unhealthy in comparison.

■ A CONSCIOUS LIVING PRACTICE FOR TODAY ■

Take a few moments to think about a key person in your life who may have resisted your attempts at change in the past. Think about whether you attempted to push or pull that person toward change with you—if so, that may be a part of the resistance you experienced. Spend time thinking of one way in which you can reassure this person that your journey of change is of you and for you, and that it is not your intention to take hostages along for the ride.

....

JUNE 6

Be thine own palace, or the world's thy jail.—John Donne

MIRRORING

If in your conscious existence you serve as a mirror to others—and, of course, to yourself—then it is no wonder that those living less consciously might not be pleased at their reflection in your joyful eyes. Even as you look on yourself with delight and newfound charm, someone else is seeing the natural reflection of the person who has not made the same commitment, who finds life and love to be an exhausting and repetitive exercise that consists mostly of making the same mistakes again and again. What does this mean for the relationships that you are in when you decide to grow, to change, to let a new way of living guide you? For the next several days, you will be considering what happens to relationships when one partner is engaged in the process of growth and change.

Look at yourself honestly and searchingly. Are you certain—in your very core—that it is not your intention to try to create change in others while publicly stating your own intention for change? This journey is about you; it is essential that you remind yourself of this along the way. Change is your own prerogative; it is not the work of others.

....

JUNE 7

The creation of a thousand forests is in one acorn.—RALPH WALDO EMERSON

BUDGETING CREATIVITY

Be sure to set aside money in your budget for creativity and creative rejuvenation. You'll know you're committed to your creativity when you systematically funnel money in its direction.

Think of your creativity as a key ongoing process in your life. It's really your most important product. If your creativity slips, everything in your life slips. Watch what happens in your life as you spend more money on your creative expression. I predict your creativity and your money supply will increase dramatically.

■ A CONSCIOUS LIVING PRACTICE FOR TODAY ■

Looking over your next week, think of a way you could invest a little extra money in your creativity. Perhaps you've been wanting a computer gadget or a paintbrush or a book of poetry. Go get it.

Then do some long-range thinking about what your creativity budget for the year might be. It's not important whether it's two dollars or two million. What matters is that you place a priority on your creativity, and support that priority with your pocketbook.

JUNE 8

Think this about the fleeting world: a star at dawn, a bubble in the stream. —BUDDHA

MAKING TRANSITIONS EASIER

Many people, including me, sometimes make our transitions harder than they need to be. Things change . . . we change . . . we all go through ages and stages and feelings—that's simply the way life is. I've learned the hard way that it helps to confide in others when I'm going through transitions. It makes the change process much easier when you can open your heart to others as you grow.

One mistake I've seen people make—and one I've made myself—is to wait until we've got things all figured out before we share them with others. Waiting until we've got things tidily wrapped and packaged means sometimes that we wait for a long time before bringing other people in on the shifts going on inside us. Dozens of times in counseling sessions I've heard an exasperated person ask something like, "Why didn't you tell me what was going on inside you?"

Make changes easier by sharing the unanalyzed experiences, the confusing things that don't make sense, the feelings that seem to have no reason for being.

■ A CONSCIOUS LIVING PRACTICE FOR TODAY ■

Find a quiet moment today to pass the following ideas through your mind:

It's all right to share my thoughts and feelings with others, even before I've figured anything out.
I don't need to understand everything I do.
I can let people in on my unanalyzed experiences.

The quality of a man's life is in direct proportion to his commitment to excellence, regardless of his chosen field of endeavor.—VINCE LOMBARDI

RESISTANCE AND THREAT

Instead of embracing your growth and change, suppose someone close to you is deeply threatened? Often this threat will express itself in one of two ways, consistent with the old "fight or flight" instinct of humans. Back in the days when our Daytimers contained lots of "bear-fighting" appointments, when we still did most of our artwork on cave walls, our bodies prepared for threat by doing one of two things: striking out at the threat (the fight response, or aggression) or running from the threat (the flee response, or passivity). Those days are long gone, and yet the human animal retains the physiological and psychological response to threat: fight or flee. If your partner seems threatened by your forward movement, and if your partner is unwilling to directly deal with this threat, you may see the conflict notching up in your relationship, or you may notice your partner creating a distance between you. *Fight or flight.* Some people, uncomfortable with a clear declaration of anger, will perform a half-fight; there will be an act of aggression, but it will be carried out in an indirect way that allows the fighter to claim no knowledge of his or her intentions. This passive-aggressive response chips away at the trust, the communication, the honesty between partners. *You stepped on my foot,* you say, sounding wounded. *No I didn't,* your partner responds, shocked that you could make such an accusation, and yet there is the bruise. What now?

■ A CONSCIOUS LIVING PRACTICE FOR TODAY ■

Fight or flight; what's your poison? Think about your typical response to stress or perceived danger (especially of the emotional kind). How does your response work for you? How does it work against you? Give some thought today to developing new ways of responding to stress.

JUNE 10

How many therapists does it take to change a lightbulb?
Only one, but the lightbulb has to want to change.—ANONYMOUS

LEADING A HORSE TO WATER

How do you have a relationship with someone who does not want to be conscious? Can you drag someone, with the proverbial kicking and screaming, into consciousness? You have undoubtedly heard the saying about leading a horse to water, and you have probably also heard the old axiom about therapy—whether an assisted process with a professional or something you set out on alone, as you are doing here—being useless unless someone *wants* help and *wants* change. There are two likely forms of resistance to change: one partner will verbally praise what you are doing and make commitments to join you in the journey toward consciousness, and yet, somehow, she or he will never seem to really be along for the ride. You will feel undermined during your travels, passivity-aggression at work. Another partner will be quite blunt about his or her unwillingness to make changes. In a sense, *this* partner is easier to deal with, because at least she or he is following a policy of honesty. Make a deep, searching examination of your partner, and give the gift of asking your partner if she or he is simply a passenger along for the ride or is planning on doing a share of the driving. If your partner wants to join you in consciousness, then you can prepare for the richness of relationship; if your partner does not, then you can continue the process on your own, deciding as you move forward whether this relationship can or will be one that allows you to be yourself most fully.

■ A CONSCIOUS LIVING PRACTICE FOR TODAY ■

Identify the one significant person in your life who is most likely to resist or attempt to thwart your attempts at change.

- How will this person be likely to resist/thwart you?
- How can you short-circuit this resistance process?

....

Relationships always bring to us the very thing that most needs our urgent attention.

GETTING MORE FAMILIAR WITH DEFENSIVENESS

One of your big tasks in the journey of conscious living is to notice all the ways you (and others) get defensive. Defensiveness slows down the creative process—it's one of the major ways you sabotage yourself when there's a possibility of a breakthrough in the air.

Here's a list of popular defensive moves: getting confused, criticizing, playing dumb, getting sleepy, getting overly busy, getting sick, reaching for a snack or a smoke, changing the subject. There are plenty more—these are just some of the common ones you can see around you every day.

■ A CONSCIOUS LIVING PRACTICE FOR TODAY ■

Imagine sitting at a stoplight, watching a very attractive person cross the street. You feel the stirring of some sexual feelings. Just then, your mate asks you, "What are you feeling right now?" The authentic response might be, "I'm feeling the stirring of some sexual feelings." If you did not have the courage to be authentic, which of the following defensive moves might you use?

Denial	Changing the subject
Playing dumb	Lying
Attacking	Making a joke

JUNE 12

What upsets me is not that you lied to me, but that from now on
I can no longer believe you.——FRIEDRICH NIETZSCHE

THE PATH OF HONESTY

Why do you long for the truth and yet spend so much energy keeping it at bay? Maybe the answer lies in your childhood, where the naked truth so often went unrewarded; you spoke from your heart and were greeted with looks of adult fury or horror or embarrassment. You, though, are committing to being truthful and to surrounding yourself with those who can bear truth. Now is the time to begin to dismantle your fear of what might happen if you make your path one of honesty.

■ A CONSCIOUS LIVING PRACTICE FOR TODAY ■

Think back to what may have happened in your past when you told the truth. The results may have been unpleasant at times. Write down a few of the outcomes that you saw as a child when you told the naked truth, and then examine these outcomes. Are you living in fear of an adult version of the very same results today?

JUNE 13

Habit is habit, and not to be thrown out of the window by any man, but coaxed
downstairs a step at a time.——MARK TWAIN

OLD HABITS

We all have habits; much earlier in this year of conscious living, you began to consider those habits that you carry with you, and that often influence your behavior. Maybe your habit is to silence your voice when conflict rears its ugly head; perhaps you have made yourself a bed out of victim-hood, one to which you retreat often and instinctively. Whatever your habit, you will have to let go of it if you are going to enter into a conscious relationship with yourself and with others. Being conscious means being aware, questioning your choices and your behaviors, not allowing yourself to lapse into the familiar and unworkable simply because it is what you have known.

■ A CONSCIOUS LIVING PRACTICE FOR TODAY ■

Think on a habit you've broken or shed. Perhaps it was physical (smoking, nail-biting, overeating), or maybe it was more of an emotional habit (avoidance in the face of conflict, for instance). Identify the habit, and then identify what helped you to let go of this unworkable habit. You can apply your success in letting go of this past habit to the methods you use for letting go of current habits you want to shed.

....

JUNE 14

Nature has given to men one tongue, but two ears, that we may hear from others twice as much as we speak.——EPICTETUS

TO LISTEN IS TO LOVE

Read the quote below on listening. I find it touching and real; the act of truly listening to another, truly engaging with another on the deepest of emotional and intellectual and spiritual levels, is a spanning of distances and a breaking down of walls. It is entering a place you have never been before, but one to which you shall forever after wish to return, and often.

Deep listening is like dying. It's a relinquishing of control . . .
a giving over into the art of what comes.

Without such an opening, conditioning stays intact,
and natural innocence disappears into an
arrogance which knows it has an answer for everything.
—TOM LUTES

■ A CONSCIOUS LIVING PRACTICE FOR TODAY ■

Make a commitment right now to deep listening. As you move through your day, let go of controlling what other people say through the grip of your automatic listening. Instead, let go and listen open-endedly, openheartedly, open-mindedly to just what people are saying.

....

JUNE 15

What we play is life.—LOUIS ARMSTRONG

EBONY AND IVORY

Laura writes: Not long ago, a friend gave an unwanted piano to my family, knowing that Timothy, my four-year-old, is a musician at heart. Tim spends hours perched on the piano bench, his small hands running gently over the keys, a virtuoso in Big Bird overalls. Several days after the piano arrived, Timothy was making music when he discovered the difference between the ivory keys and the ebony keys. I watched his expression as he pressed first a white key, then a black, experimenting over and over with the difference in sound. My little scientist had discovered something, and I waited to hear what his take on it might be. Finally, he twisted around on the piano bench and looked at me. "These ones," he said, plunking on a few white keys, "are happy. And these," he continued, striking a few black keys, "are so *sad.*" Layered on top of the major keys, the ones that range from a deep-in-the-diaphragm, rich, joyful tone to a tinkling, playful happiness, are the minor keys, which do sound sad, weighty, like warning tones or sorrowful whispers.

And such is the tone of your life; there will always be layers, a symphony of sound in which the major chords can't be separated without detracting from the minor, in which the richness of the music is directly related to the merging of good days and bad, a well dug by sorrow that ultimately leaves more room for the joy that will follow. Acceptance of the ebony and ivory of your emotional and relational lives is essential to a joyful experience of those lives.

■ A CONSCIOUS LIVING PRACTICE FOR TODAY ■

Each of you has sounds within your heart—the joyful singing when you are loving and being loved; the sad chords when you are lonely or feeling out of place in your life. Spend five or ten minutes today listening to the sounds within your heart. What are you trying to tell yourself?

....

JUNE 16
Everybody thinks of changing humanity and nobody thinks of changing himself.
—LEO TOLSTOY

SHOW ME THE FEELINGS

Certain phrases have a way of catching on in popular culture (and then disappearing, a testament to their staying power!); a year or so ago, the phrase "Show me the money!" was big. Often, these phrases catch on because they appeal to something in our culture on a larger level than that originally intended by the words. The deep suspicions and reservations exhibited by "Show me the money" are consistent with modern-day life and speak to our general distrust of checks in the mail, personnel directors who are going to call, and sincere statements of an intention to change. *I* believe in faith, though. I take people at their word when they make a commitment to change—but I don't ignore the myriad signs that such a change is not going to be forthcoming. Words are, after all, only words, and although powerful, words are not change. An intention is a positive thing, but it is not change in and of itself. If your partner says that she or he intends to change, accept the commitment on faith, and do what you can to support that growth and movement. Examine yourself and make certain that you are not standing in the way, either directly or passively. Be direct with your partner if you see signs that she or he is not living the commitment that has been made, and be unceasingly frank with yourself about your own ambivalence about this change. It is natural to feel some degree of conflict about such sweeping transition; the thing that will make this conflict manageable is if you are truthful about it, directly acknowledging and dealing with your ambivalence.

■ A CONSCIOUS LIVING PRACTICE FOR TODAY ■

Today is a day to practice making and keeping an agreement—with yourself. Decide on something for yourself, no matter how large or small, that you can make happen today. Perhaps you'll read for twenty minutes, or take a walk, or clean out those old, unwanted clothes in the closet. Perhaps you'll sit and stare into space. Make the promise and keep it, and then be aware of how it feels to honor your own agreements, to be faithful to yourself.

....

JUNE 17
He who breathes deepest lives most.——ELIZABETH BARRETT BROWNING

AN INSPIRING PROBLEM

Think of your conscious life as a breathing problem: how much can you breathe in, how much can you breathe out? In other words, regard your breathing as a metaphor for how deeply you want to live. Your full in-breath says, "I'm open to living to my deepest level of feeling," and your full out-breath says, "I'm open to expressing to my fullest in the world." Breathing is an exquisitely sensitive monitor of how you are living. At any moment your breath registers tiny fluctuations in your mood, your thinking, your surroundings. If you learn to pay attention to it, it will tell you more than the most sensitive biofeedback machine. It's no accident that many of the world's ancient languages use the words for breath and spirit interchangeably: *atman* in Sanskrit, *spiritus* in Latin, *pneuma* in Greek.

■ A CONSCIOUS LIVING PRACTICE FOR TODAY ■

As you go through your day today, tune in to your breathing now and then. Observe it nonjudgmentally: Simply notice its qualities—full, easy, hesitant, ragged, held, forced, flowing. As you notice its qualities, make connections between your breathing and what else is going on in and around yourself.

JUNE 18

Do I contradict myself? Very well, then I contradict myself.
I am large; I contain multitudes.—WALT WHITMAN

DISCOVERING YOUR ESSENCE

Great teachers of conscious living—from Epictetus to Carl Jung—have called our attention to the distinction between essence and persona. Essence is a more authentic depth of ourselves that lives beneath and beyond the various masks we use to interact with the world. That does not mean, of course, that essence is better than persona.

It's a mistake to judge persona harshly. In fact, judging our personas keeps them in place. I struggled for years in my close relationships with my "critic" persona, which took pleasure in finding fault with people. The more I tried to get rid of it, the more prominently it displayed itself. Then one day I realized the joke: I was trying to get rid of my critic by criticizing it! Of course it was never going to disappear that way. So I took an opposite tack: Loving it. Since then, it's slowly receded into the background, no longer the dragon I once tried to slay.

■ A CONSCIOUS LIVING PRACTICE FOR TODAY ■

Ask a compassionate and sensitive friend for a particular type of feedback. Explain the difference between essence and persona. Then ask: Based on your experience of me, what is my essence? What are some of my personas?

Asking for feedback is a very courageous thing to do, one of the signs of a mature person.

....

JUNE 19

Who's not sat tense before his own heart's curtain?—RAINER MARIA RILKE

SHIFTING YOUR PERCEPTION

One of the best ways to shift your perception out of habitual ruts is to ask questions of yourself. A genuine question—one that you, with all your heart, would love to have answered—can open up a wealth of learning. A friend of mine, in a moment of great humility, asked a question that immediately changed his love life. A lifelong bachelor, he had an insight one evening that his singlehood had been based on a deep fear that he could never get the kind of love he wanted. Alone in a room, he asked out loud, "How can I get the love I need?" A few seconds later he burst into tears and sobbed for a long time. A few weeks later, he met the love of his life, to whom he has now been happily married for nearly two decades.

His life became the answer to his question.

What, with all your heart, do you most want to know? What, with all your heart, do you most need to learn? What, with all your heart, do you most want to contribute?

....

JUNE 20

Everyone of us has in him a continent of undiscovered character.
—*WORDS OF LIFE*, CHARLES L. WALLIS, EDITOR

AS YOU WERE

Here is what I hope for you on your journey toward conscious love and conscious living: ecstasy, agony, joy, pain, tears, loud, hooting laughter. In other words, I hope for only the best for you; I hope for your journey to be one that takes you to the very heart of the human experience of living fully, truly, honestly. In the armed services, after a lower-level member salutes a higher-ranking member, the person of higher rank often says, "As you were," which is an instruction to return to the ease of stance that was observed before the formalities of rank intervened. Laura writes: This phrase—*as you were*—has been running through my head tonight inexplicably as I write, and by honoring it— wondering about it—I have come to understand why. I want to say to you: As you were! Return to that open, joyful, honest flow of good feeling that is your birthright, that you knew when you were too young to have learned anything else. *As you were.*

■ A CONSCIOUS LIVING PRACTICE FOR TODAY ■

Close your eyes and breathe deeply, allowing yourself to return to a time when you were you ... before expectations and disappointments and the quest for external achievement began to shape you differently.

Spend ten or fifteen peaceful moments remembering yourself as you were, and take from the memory the parts of yourself you honored and enjoyed most. How can you give those parts of yourself a stronger voice in your life today?

....

JUNE 21

Love is not love
which alters when it alteration finds.——WILLIAM SHAKESPEARE

FIRST LOVE

Laura writes: I'm remembering my first love as a teenager. I find myself thinking that I should put quotation marks around the word *love,* as if to say that I realize, being an adult, that it wasn't *really* love, that it was some adolescent approximation of love, and therefore less worthy. I stop myself and let myself remember Ted and not insult him or myself or the intensity that we shared by allowing my adult censor to rule the day. Who among us doesn't look with fondness on the rush of excitement, the stir of new sexual feelings, the intense connection that occurs in early relationship? There is a saying in the increasingly dangerous world of sexually transmitted diseases: When you have sex with someone, you also have sex with everyone she or he has slept with before. I think of this in relationship: When you love someone, you are also loving everyone you have ever loved before. You carry with you every relationship, every hurt, every joy, every pattern, somewhere imbedded in your memory. This makes your later loves heavier, at times, with the voices from the past, but also richer with experience—and it gives to your first love a lightness of being that is one of the great wonders of life.

Remember your first significant romantic relationship. Allow yourself to remember both the positive and the negative feelings you had toward the person who gave you the beginnings of your adult experience with relationship.

Spend a few moments honoring your memory and walking back through time as you think about your first love, finishing these thoughts however you wish:

She or he was _____.
Dating him or her, I felt _____.
Dating him or her made me realize that _____.
When I was with him or her, I was _____.

....

JUNE 22

Great things are done when
men and mountains meet.—WILLIAM BLAKE

YOUR HIERARCHY OF NEEDS

Abraham Maslow, a well-known psychologist, set up what he called a hierarchy of needs, which, among other things, helped to identify why certain people were engaged in certain levels of behavior. He said that before you can go on to focusing on engagement with others or self-actualization (which would include the important questions about and movement toward essence), you must first meet a host of lower-level needs, such as the need for food, shelter, and safety. Oddly, I have found the reverse to be true with essence; it is generally my experience that the more affluent the society, the greater the lack of self-knowledge. I wonder if this is because in an existence layered with things, it is harder to reach your essence. In fact, I wonder if the very purpose of the "things" people acquire isn't sometimes to provide a blockade between oneself and the difficult questions. If you allow acquisition and affluence to become a narcotic, perhaps you numb yourself enough so that the questions go away for a time. If you are out there, however, in the raw of human existence, searching for food and shelter, perhaps the questions—Why am I here? Who am I? What does this all mean?—take on a special meaning and import.

■ A CONSCIOUS LIVING PRACTICE FOR TODAY ■

Look around you at some point today when you have a moment of peace in your home. Where are you in your own hierarchy of need? Are you trying to meet the most basic level of need, food or housing? Are you focused most on safety? Or are you focused on affiliation—connecting with others? If you have managed to provide a safe haven for yourself physically and in connection with others, perhaps your energy is now directed toward self-actualization. Think about one facet of yourself that you most want to focus on and give your energy to.

Simply being present with what is has so much power that you often do not give yourself more than a split second of it.

....

JUNE 23

The great art of life is sensation, to feel that we exist, even in pain.—LORD BYRON

THE RELATIONSHIP QUESTION

One of the first things a relationship therapist learns is that couples argue to burn up energy that could be used for something else. In fact, arguments often serve the purpose of using up energy, so that the couple do not have to take the courageous, creative leap into an unknown they fear. Arguing serves the function of being a zone of familiarity into which you can retreat when you are afraid of making a creative break-through. Arguments are often like melodramas—they have a predictable beginning, middle, and end. Most couples have not had hundreds of arguments; they've had the same argument hundreds of times.

■ A CONSCIOUS LIVING PRACTICE FOR TODAY ■

Pause for a couple of minutes and give sincere thought to this question: If my closest relationships worked harmoniously and smoothly, what would I do with the energy and time now expended in conflict?

....

JUNE 24

Ask not what your country can do for you, but what you can do for your country.—
JOHN F. KENNEDY

A PURPOSE IN THE CHAIN OF LIFE

Imagine that you are a young tree being planted. See the tree in your mind's eye: the narrow, strong trunk; the reaching roots that you press gently into the soil; the limbs, some brittle and some stronger, with green buds pressed close to the bark; the new leaves that are soft and supple. Imagine your own trunk as the trunk of the tree, your arms and legs as the limbs, your feelings and thoughts as the flower buds waiting to blossom and the leaves waiting to share oxygen with the atmosphere. Like a tree, you have much to share with the world around you. You are not just decorative; you serve a real purpose in the chain of life, bringing something necessary to the environment. Let yourself recognize and accept your contributions to those around you, and if you begin to feel that you are occupying space without giving back enough, find ways to change that. It sounds like a cliché—volunteer your time, help others—but clichés gain their notoriety by being true, often. If you give back and interact with the world around you as someone who is worthy, a contributor, you will find that the world will reciprocate. A conscious life does not consist of a "me" orientation, a self-absorbed focus only on how you feel, what you want. The truly conscious person is a full contributor to and participant in the give-and-take, the ebb and flow, of the world in which she or he lives.

■ A CONSCIOUS LIVING PRACTICE FOR TODAY ■

Often on the news after a "hero story" you will hear someone say something like this: *I guess I was just supposed to be in that place at that time.*

Think of a time when you have chanced into being in the right place at the right time, somehow creating change, making a difference. Congratulate yourself for being open to the signals from the universe that guided you toward that place at that time, and think about how you can remain open in that way.

....

JUNE 25

The truth is defined as that which cannot be argued about. When the truth is expressed, there is room for the problem to transform in a healing direction.

SYMMETRY AND CIRCULARITY

There is a symmetry and circularity to life, a birth-living-dying cycle that many people spend their lives trying to outrun. We are all born, and yet so often we deny our early innocence, our dependence, the longing buried in every one of us to return to that dark, safe, pulsing ocean of the womb. We all live, and yet we so often don't really feel, experience, reach out our arms to embrace the world as a lover. And we all will die, and yet society is engaged in the most extreme campaign to outrun death ever mounted. Some of this is good—eating well, exercising, dropping the habits that call death to the door—but the emotional avoidance of the natural and necessary life cycle is denial, plain and simple. The walls you build in an attempt to keep life from catching you up in its rhythms serve only to alienate you from the realities of the human experience. If you were to admit—simple as it sounds—that you were once small and helpless, and that a part of your inner self will always feel small and helpless, and that you are now living the very life that will one day be gone, and that every day you move a step closer to the letting go of this life, what might that mean? I believe that it would mean unparalleled honesty, and that honesty, in turn, would lead you to realize that you must live *now*, not *later*; that we are all afraid sometimes, that we are all connected in the deepest of ways by our fears and our strengths and our questions . . . our humanity. Even the most deep-rooted of differences would become superficial when measured side by side against our one essential link: we are all human, and once, we all nestled in peace inside of our mother's belly, and now, we all wake up each day and look forward with a combination of hope and fear, and someday we will all return to a darkness or a light, and how we lived will be all that we take with us in the final moment.

■ A CONSCIOUS LIVING PRACTICE FOR TODAY ■

We've all heard the old adage that you can't take it with you. It's an adage because it's true. In the final moment, looking back on your life, what *do* you want to take with you? What knowledge or experience?

....

JUNE 26

From error to error one discovers the entire truth.—SIGMUND FREUD

THE ART OF BEING SLIGHTLY OUT OF CONTROL

We've all known people who were out of control—people who let their emotions gush, their bills pile up, and their waistlines go. It's never a pretty sight. A certain amount of control is important for a conscious life. So when I discuss the art of letting go of control, I'm not suggesting you get sloppy in any way. In fact, a slight letting go of control will usually make you more effective and efficient. The problem is that most of your excess control energy goes into trying to control things that you have no power over. You can't control whether someone likes you, or what happened in the past, or how the future will turn out. When you worry about whether someone likes you, for example, the amount of energy that goes into worrying is exactly the same energy that could be used to do something positive for other people.

■ A CONSCIOUS LIVING PRACTICE FOR TODAY ■

Take a few conscious breaths—slow, deep, easy. As you breathe in and out, consciously let go of controlling other people. Let them be who they are, feel what they feel, think what they think. As you move through your day, take an occasional "conscious breather," a few seconds to remind yourself to let go of controlling the uncontrollable.

JUNE 27
Whatever limits us we call Fate.—RALPH WALDO EMERSON

RETURNING TO INTENTION

An intention is one of the cornerstones of conscious living. If you will make a careful study of how intention works in yourself, you will discover a wealth of enlightenment. Think of intention as the first flow of energy in a particular direction. If you are eating a bowl of popcorn, for example, there was an original flicker of intention that sent you in that direction rather than toward mowing your lawn. There is a practical reason for studying intention. Since it occurs first, before thought and action, it makes an ideal place to catch yourself before careening into some line of thought or action that you'll later regret. If you are alone and heading toward the refrigerator late on a Saturday night, you might pause and ask yourself: Is my intention to assuage my hunger or my loneliness? A second's attention to intention can prevent an ugly moment on the bathroom scale the following morning.

■ A CONSCIOUS LIVING PRACTICE FOR TODAY ■

As your day unfolds, pause in the heat of action to ask yourself, "What is my intention right now?" Observe your intention to make sure it is driven by your unconscious programming or your chosen path of conscious living.

JUNE 28

I accept relationship itself as my primary teacher about myself, other people, and the mysteries of the universe.

LIVING AND LOVING WELL

Laura writes: At a time in my life that was chaotic, sad, and dreadfully inconvenient, and with a person who lived at a great distance, both of us having very different lives that would be nearly impossible to merge, I fell in love—a depth and breadth of love unlike anything I'd ever known—in fact, it made me rewrite my whole definition of adult love (not to mention question my sanity). The strong feelings were unexpected, immediate, total, unconditional—and one-sided: falling-down-drunk-with-love on my side, and warm affection on his, which just added to the confusion. On the one hand, I believed that this person was the one with whom I was intended to spend the rest of my life. On the other, I knew—for all the reasons above, and then some—that the relationship wouldn't continue. Life went on, as it does, and although I often think of him with fondness still, that gut-wrenching sadness is gone.

Imagine yourself being dipped in hot wax. It burns, it heals, it soft-ens—it does all of these things, some painful, some comforting. Depending on what you do with the experience, you can then harden and crack, or, if you keep warming yourself with love, you will be soft-ened again and again, turned pliable and warm and movable.

■ A CONSCIOUS LIVING PRACTICE FOR TODAY ■

I'm not sure what living well is the best revenge for, but I like the line. Let your mind go back to the warmth and excitement of a new love. Spend ten or fifteen minutes reliving the sensations, the experience, and let the glow stay with you as you go about your day today.

....

JUNE 29

Life is either a daring adventure or nothing. To keep our faces toward change and behave like free spirits in the presence of fate is strength undefeatable.—HELEN KELLER

WOE IS ME

There are those people who point to their bruises and rail against fate, insisting that a branch snapped against their tender skin, while for-getting, somehow, that they had squeezed shut their eyes so as not to see the branches ahead. "Fate," they sigh in the ever-recognizable voice of the victim. There *is* fate: floods come and tornados touch down, but imagine swimming in the raging floodwaters, letting the hungry winds of the tornado twirl you around in a wild dance of abandon. Some will hide from fate and change, cowering in the dark cellar of a frightened heart. *You, though; you are different.* You are preparing for a daring adventure of and in relationship, where you will face down fear and throw yourself right in the path of truth to yourself and others.

Find yourself a quiet place and time, and think on this: *I am different because* _____.

Are you a victim or a volunteer? Much of the pain you experience is due not to the actions of others but to how you see the world.

....

JUNE 30

Injustice never rules forever.—SENECA

WINDOWS OF UNFAIRNESS

Think back to our discussion of ten-second windows, those moments when powerful shifts occur in our lives. Some of the most important windows are those in which we are in the presence of a particular feeling. For example, you may be feeling anger, or you may be in the presence of someone who's angry.

Much anger is triggered by an instance of unfairness. Your boss comes in at quitting time and says, "Hey, don't leave. I've got something important I need you to do." It may be perfectly reasonable, yet at the same time perfectly unfair. And then a second problem occurs. Because there is often a power imbalance between people (between you and your boss, for example), you may be afraid to tell the person about your anger. So you stew in it and go home with a backache or a headache.

■ A CONSCIOUS LIVING PRACTICE FOR TODAY ■

As you go through your day, notice flickers and flares of anger. Notice whether they are in response to some unfairness. If you notice that you feel those flickers in response to unfairness, ask yourself if there is a better response you could make. Is there something you could say in the moment, for example, that would keep the anger from lodging in your body?

JULY

JULY 1

I think somehow we learn who we really are and then live with that decision.

—ELEANOR ROOSEVELT

SHAKING HANDS WITH YOURSELF

Standard therapeutic wisdom holds that each partner in a relationship must assume responsibility for 50 percent of what goes right and for 50 percent of what goes wrong. I believe, however, that each partner must assume responsibility for *100 percent of what goes right* and for *100 percent of what goes wrong.* How can this be possible, you wonder—or am I just mathematically challenged? Here is how it works: Before the existence of this relationship in your life, you were a separate entity, and, ideally, you were 100 percent responsible for your life. On a day-to-day basis, there was no one on whom you could lay the blame for the decisions you made; certainly many people ascribe their behavior and feelings to the ghosts of the past, but those people make choices to let ghosts run their lives, if so. This is not responsibility; this is victimization. Why, then, when you enter into relationship, would your behavior suddenly become the responsibility of the other? Responsibility is a celebration of wholeness. A relationship is between two or more people who are each 100 percent responsible for their lives; anything else is an entanglement. If you are more or less responsible, you are not in relationship.

■ A CONSCIOUS LIVING PRACTICE FOR TODAY ■

Take a close look at your most significant adult-adult relationship right now and estimate the degree of responsibility you take for the following areas of that relationship. It is not necessary to draw conclusions today; I will continue to work on this with you; for now, simply know your first impressions without interpretation or judgment.

- Emotional intimacy/well-being of the relationship.
- Daily chores needed to support the relationship.
- Initiation of sex and other play in the relationship.

....

Nothing in life is to be feared. It is only to be understood.—MARIE CURIE

INTERPRETING SENSATIONS

Remember a time when you were frightened, even terrified: your heart pounded and your breath caught, coming hard and fast. You have a physiological response to fear, but it is your *interpretation* of that physiological response that determines the outcome. Whether you are afraid or giddy with excitement or angry or sexually excited, many of the physical signs are similar: adrenalin rushes through your body, you sweat, your heart rate increases. You assign meaning to these symptoms because of the context. A pounding heart means a very different thing if you are alone in a dark alley rather than in bed with your lover. You can redefine your response to the fear of change.

■ A CONSCIOUS LIVING PRACTICE FOR TODAY ■

- Feel your body sensations when fear comes.
- Remind yourself that these same physical sensations are the ones you have felt during times of excitement and intense pleasure.
- Allow yourself to ride on the back of the physical sensations, letting yourself know the exhilaration of feeling strongly, intensely, instead of focusing on the context, for the moment.
- Remind yourself that what you feel is as much excitement and the thrill of the unknown as it is fear: you are allowing yourself to

live on the exhilarating side of fear without assigning it negative connotations.

....

Fust he was sick—but now he's starvin'.—JOHN STEINBECK
IN *THE GRAPES OF WRATH*

THE OPENNESS TO POSSIBILITY

At the end of John Steinbeck's *The Grapes of Wrath*, Rose of Sharon, beaten down by life—or so it appears—hungry, poor beyond your imagination, without hope, sits broken in a barn. She seems to have given up, and you can hardly blame her. But then something magical and miraculous happens; she lies down beside a starving man, who is near death. Gently pressing his head to her breast, she begins to nurse him. In the moment of greatest surrender, when she gives herself up to the awesome forces of the universe that have tried to destroy her family—floods, famines, the cruelty of property owners—she finds an answer, and her commitment to life and to the life of those in the universe around her shines through. It cannot be dimmed. I often think, in these moments, of the Chinese word for "crisis"; it is made up of the two Chinese symbols for opportunity and change. In your darkest, most hopeless times, you can be most open to change, to possibility, if you surrender yourself to complete, open relationship with the world around you.

■ **A CONSCIOUS LIVING PRACTICE FOR TODAY** ■

Spend a few quiet moments thinking about a time in your life when you have been in a state of crisis. You may want to use these beginnings of thoughts to guide you:

- The worst crisis of my life was when _____.
- I felt many things, but at the worst of the crisis, I felt _____.
- When I finally gave in to the feeling, I began to _____.
- In the time since, I have come to see that I came away from this crisis with a better sense of my _____.

When you have given yourself time to spend thinking about the crisis, make a commitment to yourself: *I commit myself to knowing and experiencing even the most difficult feelings fully so that each occasion of doubt is instead transformed into an event of wonder.*

....

JULY 4

There's only one corner of the universe you can be certain of improving, and that's your own self.—ALDOUS HUXLEY

GRATITUDE IS A SYMPTOM AND A HEALER

People feel more gratitude as they heal the wounds and disappointments of the past. I have noticed, both in my own life and in the lives of my students, that gratitude spontaneously happens the more I move through the shadows of the past out into the light of the present. So gratitude is a symptom of successful living, a sign that you are completing the unfinished business of past hurts.

Gratitude is not only a positive symptom; it's also a powerful medicine. Many times I've sat across from a person in the depths of a troubling issue, only to marvel as the person made the courageous step of expressing gratitude for the very thing that caused the wound. Rapid healing takes place when you express gratitude for something that has in the past been a source of anger or hurt for you. It takes raw courage to look your sadness, your trouble, in the eye and give it thanks for the lessons you have learned in its midst.

Take a few minutes to look around at your life. What and who are you grateful for? Say so. Write a note, stop off with a small, inexpensive gift for the object of your appreciation, or pick up the phone to share how you feel . . . and then be conscious of how it feels to be appreciating.

....

JULY 5

If you love everything, you will perceive the divine mystery in things. Once you perceive it you will begin to comprehend it better every day. And you will come at last to love the whole world with an all-embracing love.—FYODOR DOSTOEVSKY

DOSTOEVSKY'S SURPRISE

A moment from Dostoevsky's life can teach you all something important about conscious living. A political dissident in a time somewhat like our own sixties, young Dostoevsky was sent to prison by the czar. After languishing in prison for a long time, Dostoevsky was awakened one morning and marched out to face the firing squad. He and his friends were blindfolded and invited to utter a final prayer. Then the command was given to fire and . . . SURPRISE! Blanks were fired. The czar was playing a trick on them, to scare them out of their radical ways. Dostoevsky went on to write some of the greatest books human beings have produced. He became such a star that thirty thousand people turned out for his funeral. And the czar? Things didn't end as well for him.

■ A CONSCIOUS LIVING PRACTICE FOR TODAY ■

Has your life had a defining moment? Perhaps it was not as extreme as Dostoevsky's, but most of you have had turning points that shaped your life. Reflect for a moment on your defining moment. What did it teach you? How can you use it to guide you through your day?

JULY 6

It's not as bad as it sounds.—MARK TWAIN, COMMENTING ON WAGNER'S MUSIC

MUSIC TO YOUR EARS

A great friend and mentor of mine, Jack Downing, was a psychiatrist and teacher to thousands in his lifetime. Once, during a stressful time of my life, he gave me a suggestion that put me on a path I've benefited from ever since. Jack had a theory that if people put on their favorite music and danced for an hour a day, they wouldn't need therapy or psychiatric medications. This was an especially radical point of view from a doctor who'd been a standout in his field and had taught at such esteemed places as the Menninger Foundation.

I took his advice and began to do free-form movement to music whenever I felt stressed, depressed, or confused. It always had a powerful effect on elevating my mood. Soon, I was so hooked on it that I didn't wait until my mood dropped. I started doing it simply as a way to feel good, even if I didn't feel bad.

■ A CONSCIOUS LIVING PRACTICE FOR TODAY ■

Today, put a musical interlude into your day. Put on a favorite type of music, and let your body move with it. See if you can let go of any agenda other than simply enjoying the feeling of moving to music. Notice how you feel even after only ten or fifteen minutes of it.

....

JULY 7

Ownership is to fear.—SPANISH PROVERB

THE HIGH ART OF GIVING THINGS AWAY

Once, while struggling through a period of sluggish creativity, I happened to be looking in my closet for a tie to wear. Suddenly I had an insight—there were things in my closet I hadn't worn in years! They were still there because I thought someday I might need them again. This led to an even bigger breakthrough. I decided on the spot to go through my closet and take out everything I didn't absolutely love to wear. If I liked it but didn't love it, out it went. If I thought I ought to keep it (perhaps because someone had given it to me), out it went. Within an hour I had eliminated three-quarters of my wardrobe, but what was left made me feel great when I wore it. What happened immediately afterward was inspiring: overnight my creativity began flowing again. Ideas popped left and right, and the time to do my writing projects suddenly materialized. I'm sure someone out there enjoyed my clothes, because most of them were high-quality and like new. But it was really my own creativity that got the benefit of my philanthropy.

■ A CONSCIOUS LIVING PRACTICE FOR TODAY ■

Pick an area—your bookshelf, your closet, or your garage. Clear out everything you don't use. Then clear out everything you don't love. Give it away, and watch what happens in your life immediately afterward.

....

JULY 8

We make a living by what we get; we make a life by what we give.
—WINSTON CHURCHILL

AFFIRMING LIFE AND LOVE

Laura writes: On my sons' birthdays, I always pay close attention to the clock, and at their "birth moment," we have a special, quiet, intimate celebration. I set the kitchen timer and it counts down, and I describe to them, in varying levels of detail depending on age, what was happening three, four, seven years ago at this time. When the birth moment arrives, I take into my arms the birthday child and cradle him for as long as he will tolerate it, telling him that this was the moment we met, the first moment that my heart turned upside down with the rush of love of a new and perfect person entering my life. It has come to be a ritual between us, one we all look forward to. For them, it is a brief moment of return to the absolute perfection of pre-birth, and for me, it is a visit to the magic that instant, irreversible, life-changing, and life-affirming love is. The glow of the moment stays with me—and, I hope, them— long after they have run off to do other things; for hours afterward, I am bathed in the softness of new love, the intense and mythic kind of joy that we alone, as humans, can know. It is a lesson to us as adults to slow down, to savor the beginnings, to allow ourselves to return to those moments in relationship with our parents, our children, and our partners, to re-taste the sweet joy of new love in the midst of the merry-go-round that doesn't stop for such moments unless we demand that of it.

Do this: jump off the endless circling for a moment now and then and feel what it was like at the beginnings of love.

■ A CONSCIOUS LIVING PRACTICE FOR TODAY ■

Take yourself back to the moment of birth. Imagine the work that went into bringing you into the world, and the celebration that took place in the room when you drew your first breath, cried your first cry. Imagine yourself as tiny and vulnerable and new and full of hope and possibility. This new person lives within you still; access the newborn who lives within you and let yourself experience once again the momentous experience of entering the world and having the all of hope, the all of possibility, laid out in front of you.

We cannot command nature except by obeying her.——FRANCIS BACON

CARE AND FEEDING

Full-fledged summer is finally here after a long, wet, cold winter. I take a stack of paper and a pen and walk down to the reservoir. The roses are in bloom and soon their petals will carpet the bright green grass around the edges of the water. The azaleas are fully awake, bright pink and white and purple; the water itself moves with a quick, light rush. Sitting at a picnic table by the water, I watch others walking nearby, faces turned toward the sun, the water, the occasional breeze, each of us breathing in as if we have spent the winter without oxygen. When I go to write, creativity spills forth. I marvel at this as always; I marvel at the way in which my voice has grown stronger, richer, more creative since the day I decided to live in consciousness. *A little care, a little feeding,* I think, breathing deeply, taking in the summertime like a meal, watching how the lines etched in the faces around me are softened today. *It's time to wake up,* I whisper, and the sleeping world starts to stir with early dawn bird sounds and the sway of life.

■ A CONSCIOUS LIVING PRACTICE FOR TODAY ■

If you don't have an art in which you engage regularly, now is the time to find one. If you do, now is the time to commit to honoring the artist who lives in your heart. Today, identify your art, and do something—anything—to let the artist know that she or he will not starve from your neglect.

The thing that I most like to create is _____.
Today I will nurture my artist by _____.

JULY 10

Make yourself necessary to somebody.——RALPH WALDO EMERSON

AT HOME IN RELATIONSHIP

Are you at home in relationship? It is hardly uncommon for humans to move toward intimacy with others and then to back away. Fear of being known is so often the problem; you do not fear knowing another, but to let someone inside of your heart is to risk being seen as you truly are. I sometimes manage to convince myself that only I know the secrets that lie on the dark side of my heart, and the shadows there make the secrets seem frightening. Bring your secrets out into the light of day and examine them. Are they so bad? It is a form of arrogance to assume that your own secrets and thoughts are so much more weighty and dark than the secrets others hold. Be humble and know that we all are sometimes lonely, childish, selfish, petty, that we all hold onto bitterness some days as if it will keep us from drowning. The truth: every secret you hold has been held by someone else before. The truth *becomes* the truth when you acknowledge it and let it come out from its hiding place under your heart.

■ A CONSCIOUS LIVING PRACTICE FOR TODAY ■

- Go to a secret you have long held in your heart. It may be something you've said or done, or a feeling you've had about yourself.
- What quality of mine got me into this trouble to begin with? Boil this down to its essence; if you can't say it in less than ten seconds, you're not at the essence yet.
- Find the flip side of what you just identified. What about the quality has been a gift to you and to others in a different context?

The more you know yourself, the more you will forgive yourself.—CONFUCIUS

THE ACT OF A LIFETIME

If you're like the rest of us, as you grew up you found that some acts worked and some didn't. In your family, being a smart kid may have worked, while in another family a rough-and-tumble act may have gotten recognition. One teacher may have let you get away with being class clown, while another may have punished it so severely you didn't try it there. By the time you got into your teens, you had a well-established repertoire of routines that made up your personality. Adult life has a surprise for you, though: the very acts that enabled you to get recognition and avoid pain growing up become the same acts that you need to shed if you are to recover your authentic self.

There is a further surprise: you can't get rid of your acts by making them wrong. They can only be transcended by seeing them as they are—just acts—and giving them the love they need. As soon as you do that, they begin to recede in importance, replaced by your essence-self. When this happens, you can celebrate your real birthday.

■ A CONSCIOUS LIVING PRACTICE FOR TODAY ■

Take a moment right now to accept all the acts you play. Accept them just as you accept the time of day right now. As you move through the day, notice your various acts as they unfold. Accept and love them as they are.

Everything's possible with a willing mind.—ANONYMOUS

THE ART OF THE WILLINGNESS QUESTION

Learning to ask "willingness questions" can revolutionize your communications. A willingness question is a question you ask to open up a willingness on another person's part. For example, you might ask a friend, "Would you like to hear something I'm feeling right now?" or "Would you like some feedback on your article?" Many people make the mistake of charging ahead into an impactful communication without first finding out if it will fall on a receptive ear. Then they get hurt or angry when the other person doesn't receive the communication well. A willingness question can eliminate this problem.

Here are a few other examples:

- Would you like some advice on that?
- Would you like to hear an opinion I have on that?
- Would you like some information I know about that?

Always be prepared for the other person to say no. That's their right. Then you can say maybe later or okay. Chances are they'll say yes, though, and this clears the way for your communication. You still can't predict how they'll receive it, of course, but at least you've made the effort to make sure they want to receive it.

■ A CONSCIOUS LIVING PRACTICE FOR TODAY ■

Before you share your feelings, insights, or advice today, ask people if they want these communications. Ask willingness questions.

Follow your desire as long as you live.——PTAH-HOTEP

TEMPLATES IN RELATIONSHIP

The ten-second miracle is important to every person, whether at home or at work, alone or with loved ones. If you do not know a conscious move to make during the ten-second windows that create your destiny, your unconscious programming imprints these moments with your old patterns. Then these patterns recycle and escalate as the relationship proceeds. A template formed during an initial meeting of two people can produce distress decades later. Laura writes of an example: At age thirty-four, I took a twelve-day, deeply intense personal growth class; one of my classmates was a woman with whom I'd attended high school. We now lived on opposite sides of the country, and yet had ended up sitting five feet apart as we deconstructed the stories we'd created in our lives. I found myself having particular trouble letting go of this one story: When Miranda and I met in high school, I was the president of the state student council, a cheerleader, always busy, always successful, always popular. Now, sitting here with her, I found myself glossing over trouble spots in my life, insisting that I had everything under control—while tears ran from my eyes. I was allowing myself to slip back into the tired (and ineffective) old template (ever competent, never unsure) from those days. Miranda, fortunately, wasn't so easily fooled. In about eight seconds, she gently and firmly commented that it wasn't necessary for me to be competent with her—and, in fact, that she found it very distancing. Since then, we have established a friendship via e-mail that resembles something very different from that friendship we had back in the late seventies. Our words now are honest and truth-seeking, and our friendship is forming around who we are instead of around who we think others might want us to be. In a ten-second miracle, Miranda gave me a gift that continues to reverberate throughout my life: the gift of encouraging me to be myself rather than some shell that is smooth in the hand but brittle upon examination.

Like the seasonal cycles that bring us the miracles in nature, you have your own cycle. The miracle lies in reprogramming yourself to allow that which is instinctual, like honesty, to blossom in your life and relationship. The ten-second miracle is not selfish or individual; its leaves and branches are oxygen to relationship and to the self, allowing you to breathe deeply at last.

■ A CONSCIOUS LIVING PRACTICE FOR TODAY ■

Identify the feelings that serve as cues to you in a recurring, distressing pattern in a key relationship in your life.

Key relationship: _____.
Pattern: _____.
Feelings evoked (cues): _____.

....

JULY 14

This is what knowledge really is: it is finding out something for oneself with pain, with joy, with exultancy, with labor, and with all the little ticking, breathing moments of our lives, until it is ours as that only is ours which is rooted in the structure of our lives.
—THOMAS WOLFE

BEING BORN

If you have given birth to a child or have been present at a birth, you may know that first there is a stirring as the child prepares to make her journey. No one claims to know for sure what starts the birth process; scientists propose that hormones or other chemicals send signals to the mother and child, or that the uterine muscles reach some sort of medical point of reckoning. What about miracles, though? What if, instead of science, we give credit to the miracle of essence, to the human hunger for birth and rebirth, to the synergy of mother and child, with the blood flowing between them carrying the message: Now! It is time for change, for new knowledge, for life! She instinctively knows—and trusts—that it is time to become more than she already is, to start on the path toward breathing, toward knowing, toward living fully.

■ A CONSCIOUS LIVING PRACTICE FOR TODAY ■

Imagine that you are being born. This won't require a leap of faith; you have been born, and you have this memory imbedded in your very bones.

- Find a quiet, dark place in your home and lie down, curled up tightly, with your eyes closed.
- Breathe slowly and deeply, letting yourself remember the comforting sound of the waves of your mother around you, her heartbeat vibrating through you.
- Repeat this affirmation, inhaling and exhaling:

I am ready to bear myself;
I am ready to be born.

....

JULY 15

Life is to be felt, not figured out.—THOMAS HARDY

THE POWER OF EXPERIENCE

Something I learned in my first few years of practicing therapy genuinely surprised me: People's lives don't change through insight; they change through experience. For example, I've never seen an insight such as "my parents didn't love me" or "I was abused as a child" change anybody's life. What changes them is when they pause to experience their sadness about the loss or their anger at the unfairness of a situation. It's the moment of connection with experience that seems to take us off in a new and positive direction. Now I regard insight as something that sets the stage for experience. Some people become attached to insight and must be gently encouraged to let it go and open up to direct experience, such as letting themselves feel the pain of heartache or the gut-clench of fear.

■ A CONSCIOUS LIVING PRACTICE FOR TODAY ■

Ask yourself: What have I been reluctant to experience? Is there something I've been running from?

Perhaps it's a feeling such as sadness or fear. Other times it's an unfinished project or an unexpressed potential. Whatever it is, pause for a moment to let it register in your experience. Embrace it, breathe with it, open up to it.

....

JULY 16

Let him that would move the world first move himself.—SOCRATES

BREAKTHROUGHS

You can probably recall unconscious moments when something was said or done that destroyed the flow of intimacy between you and a key person in your life. Perhaps you are recalling a moment of joy and your partner cautions you that you are being overly hopeful, or perhaps your partner withdraws at your sadness in another moment. It is helpful to know that your emotional response to these reactions is linked to your earliest experiences, but it is knowing the ten-second windows that surround your response that will allow you to have conscious moments and apply the miracle moves that will change these patterns in relationship. Conscious moments are breakthroughs when you do or say something that opens a new horizon in a relationship. You step through into a new zone of possibility, one you haven't seen before. And the good news is: You are always only ten seconds away from a conscious moment.

■ A CONSCIOUS LIVING PRACTICE FOR TODAY ■

Think on a pattern that repeats itself, to your distress, in a significant relationship in your family of origin. *Determine* the ten-second window that precedes the destruction of the flow of intimacy. *Commit* to making a miracle move the next time you receive this cue. Do not engage in your normal pattern of conflict; simply stay with and honor your feelings.

The pattern: _____.
The window: _____.
The old move: _____.
The new move: _____.

....

JULY 17

I have a simple philosophy: Fill what's empty. Empty what's full.
And scratch what itches.—ALICE ROOSEVELT LONGWORTH

THE SIMPLICITY OF MIRACLES

The ten-second miracle, conscious loving, conscious living—an acquaintance listened to me talk about these ideas and said, "Easier said than done!" His comment was a gift, because by paradox, it pointed out exactly what resonates for me with these philosophies: they are simple, and saying and doing them is the same thing. They are grounded in the most natural of behaviors and thoughts; they are about being who you might have been had experience and repression and lessons that taught you to hide from yourself and others not gotten in your way. Living miraculously is about reaching the core of what is important, the very heart of your feelings and essence.

■ A CONSCIOUS LIVING PRACTICE FOR TODAY ■

Today, spend a few moments simplifying the concepts so far on your journey. Read the questions and complete them in your mind, and spend a bit of time thinking about where these statements that you make might lead you now.

- What I am learning during this stage of my journey is _____.
- What I would most like to work on learning is _____.

....

JULY 18

Take three deep breaths and call me in the morning.
—GRAFFITI ON THE WALL AT A HOLISTIC MEDICINE CONFERENCE

RELIEF IS JUST A BREATH AWAY

Remember the old advice to take a few deep breaths before making any move that scares you? It turns out that this advice is not only common sense but scientifically sound. Science now tells us that it only takes two or three deep breaths to change the anxiety chemistry in your blood in a more easeful direction. Next time you need to give a talk or take a driving test or audition for the Met, remember that you're only a few breaths away from a calmer physiology.

Popular holistic doctors such as Andrew Weil and Dean Ornish advocate breathing practices formerly found only in esoteric places like yoga classes and health spas. As medicine gets more complex and technological, many people are turning to the simplest possible treatments—moving, breathing, vibrant foods—to get the most health with the least technology.

Take three full breaths right now. Savor them. Enjoy them all the way in and all the way out. Notice what your body feels like after three full breaths.

As you move through your day, visit your internal "breath doctor" frequently. Take a few full breaths now and then to fill your body with fresh new energy.

....

JULY 19

The meaning of good and bad, of better and worse, is simply helping or hurting.
—RALPH WALDO EMERSON

EXCUSES AND EXPLANATIONS

A trap of unconscious loving that I talk about in *Conscious Loving* is the tendency to let people get away with destructive behavior in your relationships. For every destructive behavior you encounter, there is a richly textured excuse and explanation that accompanies it: *He doesn't know any better,* I hear, or *She didn't really mean to hurt me.* How is it, then, that *you* somehow know better, and why is it that despite all of those good intentions you're still hurt? In the final analysis, though, what is most important is that you design and set your own traps. It may be true that you live with a hard-hearted, no-good scoundrel—but why, then, did you choose him? And it may be so that your mother hurts you each time you interact, but why, then, do you continue to allow the interactions to take place? Conscious living means what it says: being aware of and responsible for the interactions that take place in relationship, letting go of the useless blame that changes nothing, and moving toward 100 percent responsibility, which changes all.

Identify a relationship in your life that you consider to be troubled. What about it is negative for you?

....

JULY 20

The question is this: Is man an ape or an angel?
I, my lords, am on the side of the angels.—BENJAMIN DISRAELI

THE POWER OF LEAVING ALONE

Much of the franticness you experience in your mind comes from critiquing the thoughts and feelings that flow through your consciousness every moment. Some say humans think upwards of fifty thousand thoughts a day, so things are crowded enough in your mind as it is. Then, if you add judging and criticizing those thoughts, no wonder your mind sometimes feels like Manhattan at rush hour.

What would happen if you simply let your mind be? What would happen if you just let yourself think what you think, with no attempt to edit, squelch, or control? What would happen if you let yourself feel whatever you feel? The worst that could happen is that you would just think whatever you were thinking and feel whatever you were feeling anyway.

You might find that if you leave it alone it will stop bothering you.

■ A CONSCIOUS LIVING PRACTICE FOR TODAY ■

Pause for a minute of special meditation. For sixty seconds, leave yourself alone. Take a break from wanting, doing, wishing, judging. Take a break even from accepting yourself. Just let yourself alone.

JULY 21

You become that of which you think.—THE UPANISHADS

THOUGHTS ON THOUGHTS

Here are two quotations about thoughts, drawn from teachers of conscious living from ancient times. It is remarkable that each of them says essentially the same thing—suggesting that human beings have had the same essential concerns for a long time:

Your disposition will be suitable to that which you most frequently think upon; for the soul is tinged with the color and complexion of its own thoughts.
Your life is what your thoughts make it.
—MARCUS AURELIUS

All we are is the result of what we have thought.
The mind is everything. What we think, we become.
—BUDDHA

■ A CONSCIOUS LIVING PRACTICE FOR TODAY ■

Consciously initiate several thoughts about who you want to be. Dream up a version of yourself that's pleasing. Dwell on those thoughts for a few moments, and return to them from time to time during the day.

....

JULY 22

A half-truth is a whole lie.—JEWISH PROVERB

INTEGRITY AND WHOLENESS

Integrity, from a Greek word meaning "wholeness," is widely misunderstood as a moral idea, and this misunderstanding causes people to feel ashamed to focus on integrity rather than to see it clearly. Integrity is actually primarily a matter of physics. If one of your wheels is out of alignment, it's best to think of the resulting shimmy as a matter of physics rather than morality. And that's exactly the best way to approach integrity. When you are operating with integrity, you are coming from a place of wholeness, harmony, and connection. When you are not operating with integrity, your relationship with yourself, your associates, and your organization will suffer. Eventually, the shimmy caused by lack of integrity will result in disorganization, breakdown, and failure. Integrity is the first place to look when things are not working well.

■ A CONSCIOUS LIVING PRACTICE FOR TODAY ■

Say the following sentence out loud several times, noticing how your body feels each time: *I commit to the practice of full integrity in my life.*

As you move through your day, pause now and then to say this commitment in your mind. As you encounter situations today, ask yourself how a person practicing full integrity would deal with them.

....

JULY 23

In the midst of winter, I finally learned that there was in me an invincible summer.
—ALBERT CAMUS

INTEGRITY IS BEING IN HARMONY WITH YOUR FEELINGS

Feeling is the first place you go out integrity inside of yourself. A person who does not understand feeling is doomed to operate out of integrity. A person who understands feeling is equipped with an essential skill. This anatomical fact illustrates the importance of emotion: The brain is the size of a grapefruit. The feeling portion is the size of the juicy part, while the thinking portion is the size of the rind. To make best use of your thinking capacity, you must be in harmony with your feelings. Otherwise, much of your thought processes will be taken up with noise from undealt-with feeling. Acknowledgment of your feelings—simple nonjudgmental awareness—is a key first step.

■ A CONSCIOUS LIVING PRACTICE FOR TODAY ■

Today, try on these statements, and discover if they feel true for you in your life.

- I acknowledge my anger when I'm feeling it.
- I acknowledge hurts when I feel them.
- I acknowledge fear/anxiety/nervousness when I feel them.
- I acknowledge joy/excitement/happiness (pleasant feelings) when I feel them.

Emotion = Energy Plus Motion
—ANONYMOUS

....

JULY 24

Nobody has ever measured, not even poets, how much a heart can hold.
—ZELDA FITZGERALD

EXPRESSING YOUR EMOTIONS

There are many hurtful ways to express feelings—from physical threat to rageful blame to stone-faced denial—but there are only a small number of effective ways. Effective emotional expression is the ability to communicate your feelings in a clear and straightforward way so that they are understood fully by others. Imagine being able to communicate all your feelings as clearly as you would tell someone what time it is. When you communicate the time of day, you don't need to dramatize it, hide it, or feel ashamed of it. You just say, "It's noon." It's possible to be just that clear with your feelings: "It's noon and I'm scared," or "It's three o'clock and I'm angry." Most of us are a long way from being that skilled in our emotional expression, but considering how little practice we get, we needn't feel bad. It just takes practice.

■ A CONSCIOUS LIVING PRACTICE FOR TODAY ■

Try on these statements to find out if they're true for you:

- I communicate my anger effectively.
- I communicate my hurts effectively.
- I communicate my fears effectively.
- I communicate pleasant feelings effectively.

....

JULY 25

There is more space in your body than anything liquid or solid.
—ELEMENTARY PHYSICS

FINDING THE SPACE WITHIN

You come equipped with your own powerful instrument for charting the vastness of inner space. It's called consciousness, and it comes factory-installed. All you have to do is learn how to use it.

One of the best uses of consciousness is for noticing all the levels of reality in you: feelings, sensations, thoughts, breathing, and the many facets of your personality. Solid scientific research indicates that people who know more about the various elements of themselves are not only happier, but they make fewer visits to doctors and take less medicine.

Once you decide to chart the immense regions of inner space, you'll be on a lifetime voyage of discovery.

■ A CONSCIOUS LIVING PRACTICE FOR TODAY ■

With an intention to wonder (rather than criticize or fix), place your attention on any sensation or feeling that is unarguably real inside your body. After the first sensation shifts, refocus your attention on another sensation, then another. Soon you may be able to feel the spaciousness that's behind and beneath and between all your solid and liquid parts.

....

JULY 26

He does not seem to me to be a free man who does not sometimes do nothing.—CICERO

A TASTE OF FREEDOM

In some areas of life, freedom can come from building up solid positions and defending them staunchly. That was the approach used in the Middle Ages, when castles and forts were the style. However, in close personal relationships, this strategy never seems to work very well. Perhaps building walls and moats around you can keep out invading hordes of barbarians, but, as Sally Kempton says, "It's hard to fight an enemy who has outposts in your own head." In most of real life, and certainly in intimate life, freedom comes from letting go of your positions, in letting go of defending them.

The moment you realize that there's nothing to defend, suddenly there's nothing to defend against.

■ A CONSCIOUS LIVING PRACTICE FOR TODAY ■

Take a close look today at your defensive patterns. Notice, as you go through the day, what your positions are and how you defend them. Notice that most of them were built to defend you against things that no longer exist in your life.

JULY 27

You can see a lot by just watching.—YOGI BERRA

THE FLICKER AND FLOW OF BODY SIGNALS

All of you are involved in the intricate play of human communication. Many of you overlook its hidden treasures, though, and suffer as a consequence. You miss the flicker of an eye-shift that could have helped you understand a key emotion in a beloved, or the nervous gesture that might have helped you determine why your sales pitch wasn't going well.

The genius-level healers of the present and past—people such as Sir William Osler, Virginia Satir, and Milton Erickson—made it clear that their skill rested on the keen observation of subtle body signals more than on any other technique. Osler once said that if you were sensitive to patients' body language, they would not only reveal the illness but show precisely how it must be treated.

■ A CONSCIOUS LIVING PRACTICE FOR TODAY ■

Today in your conversations, notice the shift of energy patterns as signaled by body language. Pay particular attention to eyes, hands, and mouth. For example, you might ask an employee if she can meet a deadline. As you do so, you notice her eyes blink rapidly and her brow creases. Regardless of whether she says yes or no verbally, it's her body communication that must be heard. Don't be afraid to ask things like "I noticed your eyes blink and your brow crease—what were you feeling when I asked you about the deadline?" People will usually be glad you're that sensitive.

I'm not crazy about reality, but it's still the only place to get a decent meal.
—GROUCHO MARX

WHAT'S FOR BREAKFAST?

A powerful businessperson told me once, "Wheaties are great, but feedback is the real breakfast of champions." He went on to say that every successful person he'd ever met was skilled at taking feedback. Check out this piece of wisdom in your own life. Hasn't your success and happiness grown hand in hand with your ability to receive feedback?

One of the hallmarks of a conscious life is the ability to give and particularly to receive feedback. Yet very little training is given in traditional schooling on these crucial skills. Make your life an experiment in learning to give and receive significant feedback.

■ A CONSCIOUS LIVING PRACTICE FOR TODAY ■

Start by making a personal commitment: *I commit to receiving feedback with gratitude and enthusiasm.*

As your ability to receive feedback grows, you may wish to deepen that commitment: *I commit to going out each day in search of meaningful feedback.*

....

Just one great idea can completely revolutionize your life.—EARL NIGHTINGALE

AN UNFLINCHING GAZE

In order to evolve along the path of conscious living, it's necessary to develop an ability to look unflinchingly at any ways in which you're out of integrity. This skill becomes more important the faster you move in life. A misaligned wheel on an oxcart doesn't cause much of a problem, but a slightly-out-of-integrity wheel on a Grand Prix racecar can spell death and destruction.

It behooves any traveler on the path to check for misalignment frequently. The quickest way you get out of truth with yourself is to bend, fold, or mutilate the truth when you speak. Be careful even in telling social lies: If you're angry and say you're not, you set up a force-field of dishonesty around you. If you say you'll call someone later and you don't, the field enlarges. Soon it can precede you wherever you go, and linger after you're gone.

■ A CONSCIOUS LIVING PRACTICE FOR TODAY ■

Renew your commitment to authentic speaking today. Do your best to avoid putting even the subtlest spin on the truth.

....

JULY 30

Facts do not cease to exist because they are ignored.—ALDOUS HUXLEY

SPEAKING FROM THE CONTEXT OF DISCOVERY

Notice that every sentence that springs out of your mouth is from one of two contexts: discovery or defensiveness. In other words, when you speak a sentence, the words make a vibration in the air that floats over to the other person's ear on an invisible raft of context. Imagine yourself feeling a racy, queasy feeling in your stomach while engaged in an emotionally charged conversation. Perhaps you'll notice the other person's gaze wandering off.

Instead of saying, "You're not listening to a word I say," which would spring from the context of defensiveness, speak from the context of discovery. Say something like, "I just noticed your gaze shifting off," and "I'm feeling racy, queasy feelings in my stomach. As I tune in to it, I think I'm afraid. I'm wondering how we can communicate here." This kind of communication may sound strange at first, but after a while you'll get more skilled so it will sound insightful rather than artificial.

■ A CONSCIOUS LIVING PRACTICE FOR TODAY ■

As you go through your day today, notice the context of your spoken communication. Notice the words other people speak to you and to each other. Simply observe the context and notice whether it's discovery or defensiveness. You may be surprised, as others have been, at how much of the latter you observe.

....

JULY 31

There is no limit to the amount of self-acceptance we need.—ANONYMOUS

A NEW LEVEL OF ACCEPTANCE

Here is a new way to feel the power of acceptance. It's a "trick of the trade" taught in training programs for therapists so they will know how to help their clients feel acceptance.

Notice what it feels like to accept what day it is today. For example, suppose today is Friday. Feel how you can accept that. In your mind, think, "Today is Friday and I accept it." Repeat this sentence a few times in your mind. At the moment you say the day, notice in your body what it feels like to accept whatever day it is. By contrast, imagine how it might feel to resist accepting that it's Friday. Your body would feel completely different inside, even though it wouldn't change the fact that it's Friday. You're going to apply this, of course, to more difficult concepts, but for now I want you to simply focus on how it feels to accept that which is unarguably true.

Now, use this same technique to accept something real that you haven't been able to accept. For one person it's something about the past that can't be accepted; for another it's something about a body part; for a third it might be an unbearable loss. Focus on one of your biggest problems. For example, say, "It's Friday and I'm thirty pounds over-weight," or, "It's Monday and I really hate my job," or, "It's Saturday and I can't control my drinking." Until you can accept reality exactly as it is, you cannot change.

AUGUST

No inquiry on the inner plane is useful unless it translates to improved action, even social action, in the outer world.

WORRY NEVER GETS YOU ANYWHERE

People often are shocked when they find out the real reason for worry: it keeps you from having to take effective action. Many of you think that if you worry enough, some good will come out of it. Usually what happens is that you worry yourself into exhaustion, which causes you to let go of control long enough for some kind of more positive outcome to occur. The worry part can be eliminated—go directly to letting go.

You'll find that the worry was not a necessary part of the process. It was just noise created by your mind because it couldn't figure out a better technology. Next time you notice yourself worrying, try out a new technology, the "wonder question." A wonder question begins with the words *I wonder* and asks a question you genuinely don't know the answer to.

Maybe you are worrying about whether you have enough money to pay all your bills. Stop the worry stream and introduce a wonder question: "How can I always have plenty of money to do all the things I want to do?"

■ A CONSCIOUS LIVING PRACTICE FOR TODAY ■

As you move through your day, nip your "worry thoughts" in the bud and turn them into wonder questions. See how many wonder questions you can generate by the end of the day. Notice at the end of the day how much lighter you feel.

AUGUST 2

What is the use of running when you are on the wrong road?——ANONYMOUS

TAKING FUN SERIOUSLY

Fun has a bad rap, because many people think of it as something trivial, a matter of video arcades and bowling alleys. Fun is definitely neglected as a valid path of enlightenment. Many people think that seriousness and suffering are the hallmarks of psychological and spiritual growth. In fact, I believe that the opposite is true. No path of conscious living is of value unless you have more high-quality fun as a result of it. I have had the pleasure of being around many great teachers of conscious living, both famous and obscure, and almost all of them were funny. Some were so off-the-scale wildly funny, in fact, that the people who couldn't handle their humor fled in dismay.

■ A CONSCIOUS LIVING PRACTICE FOR TODAY ■

Seek fun first in a good dictionary. Look up the word and its origins. Find out which definitions you like best. Determine for yourself what fun is, and find out whether you could make it part of your journey today.

....

AUGUST 3

Wonder, rather than doubt, is the root of our knowledge.——ABRAHAM HESCHEL

MASTERY OF CONFLICTS

When any problem arises, make the three following related moves as quickly as you can. Each produces instant results; all three together speed up the flow of miracles. First, take ownership of the issue itself. If you're in an argument or difficult situation, say, "I claim full responsibility for creating this argument or situation." This puts you in the power position. Second, take ownership of the (unconscious) intention that's working. Say, "I must have a need to create an argument with you right now." Third, take ownership of the solution. Say, "I take responsibility for creating a favorable outcome." Do not under any circumstances let the other person's reaction dictate how you proceed. The core ingredient in the mastery of conflict? Wonder, not judgment. To wonder about your own responsibility allows you to move forward in relationship.

Laura writes: I was once talking to a male friend, sharing a feeling I often had at the time that men didn't listen to me. When I stopped talking, I noticed that my friend had a blank look on his face. I questioned him, and he admitted that he had "zoned out" and hadn't heard much of what I'd said. In the past, I'd have taken a victim role ("Poor me! This just confirms what I was saying!"). Instead, since that hadn't worked, I looked at how I might be looking for men who didn't listen, and I examined whether I was talking in a way that made listening difficult. The answers I found in myself were quite telling, and I began to make some long-needed changes in how I sought out relationships with men. Had I stayed in the old templates, refusing to take ownership of my role in the dynamic, I'd still be back where I was, taking cold comfort in being a victim.

■ A CONSCIOUS LIVING PRACTICE FOR TODAY ■

Reflect back over the watershed experiences of your life, both in the positive and negative sense. How long did it take you each time to claim full responsibility for creating the experience? Are there some experiences you still have not claimed ownership of? If so, what are you waiting for?

Before initiating any significant conversation, pause for a few seconds to cultivate a feeling of genuine appreciation for the other person. Once attained, speak the truth of this as your lead-in to whatever else you want to discuss.

AUGUST 4

As we acquire more knowledge, things do not become more comprehensible
but more mysterious.—ALBERT SCHWEITZER

SYSTEMS OF LOGIC

In a conflict, you'll often notice that the methods you use to persuade or convince someone of something follow three basic approaches. If you use *Western logic*, you'll use facts, statistics, and evidence to make your case. If you use *theological logic*, you'll try to persuade another by discussing the morality, the right and wrong, of behaviors and choices. And if you use *Eastern logic*, you'll tend to approach behavior and choices from a stance of fate, a "que sera, sera" (what will be, will be) approach. Listen in on someone's conflict and try to identify which form of logic is being used—and then notice if the logic is being applied to feelings. You may sometimes find yourself in what I call (with tongue firmly in cheek) "a litigation of love," wherein you try to convince another of the validity and reasonableness of how you feel, as if feelings require shoring up and proof. In truth, however, feelings are fact, stand-alone realities that neither require evidence nor lend themselves to proof or debate. In conscious relationship, an essential goal to move toward is reaching a place where you no longer feel the need to defend your feelings, and also reaching a place where you do not demand proof from another about the validity of what the other feels.

■ A CONSCIOUS LIVING PRACTICE FOR TODAY ■

Store this knowledge and affirmation away for your next conflict: *My feelings are facts.*

In your next conflict with a partner, remind yourself of this affirmation, and do not allow yourself to provide evidence (i.e., examples that support your contentions) that your feelings are valid. Simply describe your feeling(s) and leave it at that.

To everything there is a season:
a time to laugh, a time to cry, a time to live, a time to die.——ECCLESIASTES

GRIEF AND THE GREAT DIVIDE

You all suffer loss, and for most of you, the losses become more frequent as you get older; first you watch as a generation twice removed begins to meet with death, and then, the generation just before your own ages and begins to encounter mortality. As you watch the chipping away of this last mountain that stands between you and your own mortality, you can experience a host of feelings, not the least of which is terror. Is there a way to meet mortality—that of those you love and that of yourself—in a way that is more conscious, that gives voice to the terror while coming to an acceptance that allows the feelings to recede?

There is. The answer is surprisingly simple: in the course of making a commitment to conscious living, your grief and your loss become less about pain and more about how much resistance you put forth to that which simply *is*, to *reality*. Consciously experiencing life—and death—is about coming to accept that there is both a flow *and* an ebb to the universe—a reason, if you will, for all things, even those that most grieve and perplex you.

For the next five days I will discuss loss, and the stages that you go through when faced with loss. Grief is, at once, the most highly personal and the most similarly played out of human experiences. Join me as I walk through a time of grief; allow yourself to re-experience your own losses, and to begin to love the place in yourself that has been made for, and of, the large and small losses that we all must know.

■ A CONSCIOUS LIVING PRACTICE FOR TODAY ■

Think for a moment of the greatest loss you have experienced. Perhaps it was the death of someone near to you, or perhaps the ending of a relationship. Let yourself experience again the feelings you knew when the loss was most fresh, most raw; these feelings are necessary to loss, and necessary to love.

....

AUGUST 6

Let my heart be wise. It is the gods' best gift.——EURIPIDES

A STATE OF GRACE

When I was younger, I had a prayer or an affirmation that went something like this: *Please give me* _____ *(whatever it is I want).* Whether it was a job or a lover or a financial windfall was largely irrelevant; I asked that the universe adapt itself to my wishes and desires. As I gained more age and experience, my prayers and affirmations changed, and whether you believe in a deity, fate, or some other force—perhaps a combination of personal will and the randomness of fate—that determines the larger outcomes in your life, I encourage you to consider the content of your requests of the universe.

A conscious life means living in a state of grace in which you recognize and accept that you have tremendous influence on and responsibility for that which happens in your life—and recognizing and accepting that there are times when your wishes are not fulfilled, and that the universe has a reason for disappointing you. You cannot know the master plan, or perhaps there is no master plan at all; you can only live your life consciously and responsibly, and then you must surrender to the grace of accepting reality as it is, not as you would sometimes wish it to be.

■ A CONSCIOUS LIVING PRACTICE FOR TODAY ■

When you are most in conflict with reality, wishing most for things to be as they are not, repeat this affirmation to yourself: *My greatest wish* is to live in a state of harmony and grace and to gracefully and lovingly accept that which I cannot change.

....

Wisdom comes alone through suffering.—AESCHYLUS

RECONSTRUCTION

A woman I know who is in her eighties recently had a facelift, believing that restoring her youthful appearance would also restore the happiness she remembers from an earlier time in her life. At around the same time, her great-niece, a woman in her twenties, underwent liposuction to remove cellulite and fat from her hips and thighs. The younger woman's hopes were similar to those of her much-older aunt; she was convinced that she would find love and be happier once her body matched an imagined ideal. A year of so after the surgeries, I had the opportunity to speak separately to each of the women, who did, indeed, both look different.

The older woman showed us the tiny scars hidden in her hairline, and she bitterly remarked on the somewhat odd perpetual smile she now wore as the result of the tightness of her skin. "I wasn't happy before the surgery," she said sadly. "And I just *look* like I'm happy now."

The niece showed off her new figure and said she still hadn't met the man of her dreams. "I suppose men look at me more now," she sighed, "but looking isn't touching. So far, nothing has changed."

You can tighten, you can remove the excess; it is a truth in our medical-miracle society. Better to loosen up the sadness blocked inside first, though, or slowly carve off the behaviors and walls that make you seem unapproachable.

Focus on the part of your body you most often wish was different. Close your eyes now and love that part of yourself. Love the roundness of your hips, the softness of your skin, the you that is the part of yourself that most needs your loving acceptance.

....

AUGUST 8

The eye is the jewel of the body.——HENRY DAVID THOREAU

DENIAL: THE FIRST LINE OF DEFENSE

Elisabeth Kübler-Ross, the author of *Death and Dying* and the scholar who first introduced the world to the stages of grief that we all experience, identified five typical stages to loss. The first stage, *denial,* occurs when a loss is first experienced. Whether the loss is the death of a loved one, a diagnosis of illness for ourself, or any other severe trauma to our life, most of us tend to initially enter a state of denial: *This can't be! I don't believe this! I refuse to accept that this is so!* While even the most conscious among you does not reach out your arms, grinning, to embrace bad news, your initial reaction to loss or potential loss can color every moment that occurs from that point on in the grieving process. A strong faith—whether in a God or fate or a set of rules that you live and love by—helps to short-circuit the process of denial. While I do not enjoy loss, I accept it; I recognize that loss is no less a part of the greater plan of the universe than is love, and that the more love and connection I experience with others, the more loss I stand to experience when I lose loved ones, through death or distance.

Consciously living out the experience of loss means starting at a place of acceptance, preparing yourself well before your first loss for the eventual, unavoidable loss that will occur. We all live—some more than others—and we all die. It is a fact of the universe, and the denial, the tightening of your heart and mind against the inevitable, is part of what creates such tremendous pain in the experience of loss.

■ A CONSCIOUS LIVING PRACTICE FOR TODAY ■

Think again, as you did yesterday, of the greatest loss you have experienced. Remember your initial reaction. How did denial manifest itself? Below is a list of the three typical ways in which we experience denial. Think for a few moments today about the ways in which you experienced denial, and an alternative had you lived in acceptance.

- Physical denial: _____.
- Mental denial: _____.
- Emotional denial: _____.

AUGUST 9

Anger as soon as fed is dead—
'tis starving makes it fat.—EMILY DICKINSON

ANGER: FIGHTING BACK

The second typical stage of grief is *anger*. This tends to occur when you are moving out of the denial that is your first line of defense; I suspect that the knowledge of the emotional pain to come tends to infuriate many people. With loss comes a reminder of the extent to which you lack control over the universe, and many people do not take kindly to the experience of losing control.

However, if you rewrite the script from the genesis of your grief, experiencing denial as acceptance, the anger that is such a common stopping point is unlikely to occur to the same extent. This is not to say that you may not feel angry at all; I can certainly imagine feeling fury at the selfishness of the suicide victim who damaged her children, or rage at the teenager who drank a great quantity of alcohol before wrapping his car around a tree, thus setting in motion tremendous grief for his parents. This anger, however, is well placed; the typical rage of grief is a vague and murky cover for sorrow, a wall you build around your sadness so that you will not have to experience grief (it doesn't work, of course; it simply holds the sorrow at bay for as long as you maintain the fury).

Thus, if you start at acceptance, you find yourself next moving to a place of sorrow, bypassing the rage that can stick in your throat, damage your heart, create havoc in your life. You drop down below rage to the sadness that almost always makes the foundation for anger (it is my experience that real rage is a rare thing; almost always, anger is a replacement emotion for loss and grief). Since you must eventually reach sadness anyway, why not bypass the unproductive anger?

■ A CONSCIOUS LIVING PRACTICE FOR TODAY ■

What did you lose when you experienced your greatest loss? It may be helpful to you to tell yourself the truth about that for which you grieved.

I told myself I was angry about/at _____.
In truth, I was grieving because I lost _____.

....

AUGUST 10

Man goeth to his long home, and the mourners go about the streets . . .
—ECCLESIASTES 12:5

BARGAINING: A DEAL WITH THE DEVIL

The third typical stage of grief is *bargaining*. It goes something like this: if things can be restored to the way they were before, I will

_____ (appreciate the deceased more, quit smoking, never say an angry word again, tell only the truth, and so on). If your *anger* is in response to the universe's reminder about the extent to which you lack control, *bargaining* is your attempt to regain a sense of control over the universe.

You have been rewriting your script, though, by experiencing denial as acceptance, and thus experiencing your anger for what it truly is: grief. The result? Less of a need to bargain with the universe, since you have already accepted reality. If you accept that there are reasons for the things that occur, even those things you least understand and that cause you the greatest sorrow, you are unlikely to experience the urge to try to control the master plan. What is, *is*.

In this world of Western logic, we often rail against the more Eastern mind-set, which is fate-based. I would recommend giving the Eastern approach a try. This is not to say that you are without responsibility, without impact on the world around you. To the contrary. Instead, I am simply saying that once something takes place, it *is*. It is no longer negotiable, and to the extent that you can let go of your need to try to rewrite history, you will be living in more of a state of synchronicity and acceptance with the universe.

■ A CONSCIOUS LIVING PRACTICE FOR TODAY ■

Again focusing on your greatest loss, do you recall any bargains that you tried to strike? What were they? When you realized that your bargaining would not change the course of events, how did you feel?

The bargains I tried to make were _____.
When my bargains didn't work, I felt _____.

AUGUST 11

And you wonder where we're going,
where's the rhyme, where's the reason?—JOHN DENVER

DEPRESSION: WHEN BARGAINING FAILS

When bargaining fails to work, as it inevitably will (try controlling the universe; you'll notice that it is notoriously resistant to your attempts), *depression* can set in. It is my belief that this depression is the answer at which people most often arrive when faced, in one experience, with both loss and a sense of their own helplessness. If you recall, though, that your helplessness is because of the futility of your attempts to control that which cannot and will not be controlled, you have tremendous power, then, to change your experience of grief— and again, it all goes back to that initial processing of your loss. It all goes back to acceptance of reality.

Letting go, letting *acceptance* rather than *resistance* rule your experience of life—and loss—you become a part of the machinery of the universe rather than a wrench thrown into the works. The wrench never stops the wheel from turning for long; in the end, it is spit out, damaged and changed. You must refashion yourself so that you no longer need to be the wrench; instead, you must see yourself, even at the worst of times, as an integral piece of the puzzle that surrounds you. The fact that there are times when you do not understand the rhyme or reason of the puzzle does not mean that you are not part of it. Better to be a part of the universe, unable to see its whole at times because you are in the middle of it, than standing on the outside, trying to stop it from being what it is.

■ A CONSCIOUS LIVING PRACTICE FOR TODAY ■

What finally allowed you to begin to move past your deep sorrow? As you look back now, can you see ways in which you prolonged your sadness by your resistance of it?

I am going to seek a great Perhaps.—FRANÇOIS RABELAIS'S DYING WORDS

ACCEPTANCE: THE PATH TO ETERNITY

Laura writes: One day in the halls of a university, I overheard a public-speaking student talking to a friend. He was explaining to the friend how one writes the proper eulogy. "You gotta acknowledge the death, acknowledge the life, acknowledge the grief, help people accept it, yada yada yada," he said. I laughed at his somewhat callous and calculated methodology for helping people deal with loss, and yet the more I thought about, the more I realized that he was right, at least from a technical standpoint. All good eulogies I've heard met the exact criteria he identified. And what it comes down to is that they're all about the acceptance of reality, the acceptance, as Gay has said, that what is, *is.*

And here, in what is the fifth stage of the typical grief response, I come to *acceptance,* to what I intuitively believe should be your first and most important work when confronted with loss. Acceptance.

I believe that it is important to write this reminder: I am not suggesting that sorrow and a sense of loss and a sense of rage at your loss is abnormal or wrong or bad. I, too, have experienced great loss, and will continue to do so, I know, throughout my life. I have not danced or clicked my heels or sent shouts of joy to the heavens during times of loss; I have probably done what you have done: asked why such pain is necessary, and tried to duck and dodge the sorrow. What I have learned, though, is that railing against fate, demanding that the wheel stop turning or that time reverse itself or refusing to accept reality only prolongs my experiencing of loss and distances me from the very universe that can comfort me in its hugeness and its depth.

As you look back now on your greatest loss, have you accepted what happened? If you have, how did you reach acceptance? If you have not, what is one thing that you can do today to move yourself forward in your journey?

....

AUGUST 13

Never, "for the sake of peace and quiet" deny your own experience or convictions.
—DAG HAMMARSKJÖLD

CONVENIENTLY FORGETTING

Do you know someone who makes agreements—large or small—that she or he does not keep, and then insists that she or he simply forgot? Or is this your own relational habit at times? When you hear yourself or another saying, "I forgot," it is a relationship warning to rival bells and alarms and great clanging noises. We all forget—we are human, after all, and hardly corner the market on perfection—but when you forget agreements, except in the most rare of instances, it is a signal of something greater, something more personally damaging than a simple slip of the mind.

To be conscious is to remember. You can carry this out in any number of ways—remembering can be a complex skill, and you may wish to use multiple methods for remembering and carrying through on the agreements you make. The key, however, is in the commitment, in the motivation. If it is truly your wish to have a conscious relationship, you must fully commit yourself to remembering the agreements you make, and then to keeping those agreements.

When you say, "I forgot," what you are really saying is, "It wasn't important enough for me to remember." Take heed; it is a message no one wants to hear.

Remembering can be complicated by your mental, psychological, and emotional states; it can be affected by what is going on in the environment and by how an agreement is phrased. Help yourself keep your agreements by using any or all of the following methods to increase retention:

- Visualize the agreement; see it as a picture, a part of your partner.
- Repeat the agreement out loud to your partner to reinforce it.
- Link the agreement to other beliefs that you already follow through on.
- Ask your partner to assist you with a gentle reminder at times, if you can do so without turning the responsibility for keeping the agreement into your partner's problem.

....

AUGUST 14

I must create a system,
or be enslaved by another man's.——WILLIAM BLAKE

RESPONSIBILITY

Read the very last line of the previous exercise. It is a recommendation for how to better remember agreements you've made, and it says: *Ask your partner to assist you with a gentle reminder at times, if you can do so without turning the responsibility for keeping the agreement into your partner's problem.* There are times when your partner fails to keep agreements, and then turns to you in anger and says, "But you didn't remind me!" Perhaps you have heard these words come from your own lips. If so, it is time for you to look at the degree to which you or your partner is truly being 100 percent responsible for agreement-keeping in your relationship. It is not harmful to ask a partner for a reminder at times; this is how a partnership works. However, ultimate responsibility for what you do—and for what you fail to do—rests with you and with you alone. It is always remarkable to me that people who are capable of holding down highly responsible jobs—an attorney, say, or a medical doctor—proclaim themselves as being incapable of remembering a partner's birthday, or remembering that Thursday is garbage night. An adult, someone who is taking 100 percent responsibility for what he or she brings to relationship, recognizes that *agreement-keeping is a choice*, plain and simple.

■ A CONSCIOUS LIVING PRACTICE FOR TODAY ■

Rather than leave agreement-keeping to chance, dive into your agreements with your eyes open and your heart committed. When you make an agreement with a partner, regardless of the size or complexity of the agreement, state it out loud. You can't commit halfway to consciousness and agreement-keeping; simply saying the words doesn't count. You have to walk the talk: *I promise to take out the garbage on Thursday nights. I will keep this agreement with you.*

....

AUGUST 15

There is no saint without a past, no sinner without a future.
—ANCIENT PERSIAN MASS

PERSONAL STYLE

You are the neatest person on earth—even your socks are filed away by color and style—and your partner is having a good day if she or he manages to remember to *wear* socks. Or perhaps it's the reverse. When does behavior stop being about personal style and start being about irresponsibility?

The first thing to consider is that you chose your partner, socks and all. To come back at your partner after the fact and demand change raises the question of how realistic you were being early on. Ideally, you would all have the insight to fully consider the long-term effects of your behavior and your partner's behavior when you form a relationship, but age, experience, and life changes make this somewhat difficult. At twenty-five, single and childless, it is hard to know how your partner's parenting style will influence your daily existence.

For today, let's focus on accepting your partner fully, recognizing that she or he is human, after all, and though undoubtedly less perfect than you, perhaps not so bad after all.

■ A CONSCIOUS LIVING PRACTICE FOR TODAY ■

Think about your partner for a moment, considering what drew you to him or her to begin with. Think about the three things you most liked about your partner early on, and then think about the three things that now cause you the most trouble with your partner. See any connections? You are likely to, if you look closely. It is often that which you most admire in your partners early on that causes you the most grief over the years. For today, there is no need to do anything about this; simply know it.

....

AUGUST 16

Utter originality is, of course, out of the question.—EZRA POUND

THE OYSTERS-IN-THE-STUFFING DILEMMA

Yesterday, you focused on acceptance of your partner regardless of the differences between you, and regardless of your possible belief that your way is, indeed, superior to your partner's. Today, let's look at that hidden or not-so-hidden belief that *your* way is the *right* way.

Have you ever gone to a Thanksgiving dinner at someone else's house? Where was the broccoli casserole? The sweet potato pie? Could those have been *oysters* in the stuffing? It is distressing when people do things differently than you do. You are raised in a certain environment, doing things a certain way; to adapt yourself to and compromise with another's style can be one of the trickiest parts of a long-term relationship. It is also one of the keys to making it work over the long haul.

What danger lies in giving up your superiority? What might happen if you acknowledged that you do not corner the market on the right or the moral way to live a life, except for your own?

■ A CONSCIOUS LIVING PRACTICE FOR TODAY ■

Call to mind a simple conflict you have had with your partner about how something should be done. Perhaps it is a conflict about what clean means, or perhaps it is related to holiday traditions or child-rearing styles. As you think about the conflict, also think about identifying three simple ways that you can accept and respect your partner's style and approach without letting go of your own.

....

AUGUST 17

Out of intense complexities, intense simplicities emerge.—WINSTON CHURCHILL

RESPECT AND HOSTILITY

Laura writes about stopping at a convenience store recently: Opening my car door, I accidentally bumped the next car over. I got out and checked for damage and was relieved to find that there wasn't so much as a smudge on the other car. Going inside on my errand, I was verbally accosted by a woman who yelled at me about the damage I had caused to her car and, worse, about how obvious it was that I didn't care about the damage as long as I thought no one saw me cause it. Perplexed (since

I *had* checked the car, and very much *did* care), I asked the woman to show me the damage; the woman fumed and blustered, but since she was still inside the store and hadn't looked at her car yet, she was obviously unable to do so when we walked outside together.

"You people in your expensive cars think you own the world," the woman growled as a parting shot as she drove away. I looked at my car with new eyes (it's not in the luxury class, I can assure you) and then watched as the woman screeched tires out of the parking lot. I was deeply upset by the encounter, and drove to a nearby park to think about what had happened. I felt a sense of outrage at the accusations that had been made, and unsettled by the amount of hostility that had been directed at me. As I sat in the park, a realization settled over me: "You people" must have been made up of a huge list of grievances committed over time. For whatever reasons, I represented the hostilities with which this woman had felt targeted. By putting myself in her place as best as I could, and trying to understand the world from her angle, I was able to let go of my outrage and join her in her own. I tasted the lack of respect she was carrying around on her shoulders like a heavy cape in summer. This allowed me to locate an empathy and comprehension within myself that I would not otherwise have been able to reach. That, in turn, allowed me to let go of my own upset.

■ A CONSCIOUS LIVING PRACTICE FOR TODAY ■

Next time you are the target of hostility, take a moment to remove yourself from your own experience. Put yourself into the experience of the other, asking yourself these questions:

- What feelings is the other person having right now?
- What experiences might have contributed to this person's hostility?
- How might I feel/behave if I had had the same experiences as this person?

He who wants a rose must respect the thorn.—PERSIAN PROVERB

BREAKING OUT OF THE PRISON OF IDENTITY

In the journey of learning to live consciously, you may find, especially if you've reached midlife, that the very identities that enabled you to become successful have to be let go so that your deeper self can emerge. I got my Ph.D. in 1974, and, after doing the required thousand hours of supervised internship, I received my clinical psychology license. By doing these things, I became qualified to assume the identity of "psychologist." Although I was proud of this identity, and it enabled me to help many people, eventually I found that it had a downside. Because I was now a doctor and an authority figure, it became more difficult to relate to people simply as human beings. Because of my identity, I had to struggle not to see people in terms of their problems. I found that to become the kind of therapist I wanted to be, I had to see through my identity so I could connect with people purely on universal human terms. The process—of letting go of my professional identity so I can be the professional I want to be—continues every day.

■ A CONSCIOUS LIVING PRACTICE FOR TODAY ■

Ask yourself: What are my treasured identities? What are their values? What are their costs? How can I hold my identities in such a way that I become most authentic?

The tragedy of life is not so much what men suffer, but rather what they miss.
—THOMAS CARLYLE

MOOD RINGS

You may or may not be old enough to remember the phenomenon of mood rings. They hit the market in the 1970s, right around the time of earth shoes and pet rocks, if I recall correctly. The concept with mood rings was that you wore the ring and it changed color based on your body temperature, indicating your mood by the color of the stone in the ring. When the stone turned green, you were happy; if it was red, you were angry . . . and so on. I was never quite sure how the thing worked, but it made a good conversation-starter, if nothing else.

What if you could put on something that reversed the process? What if you could put on a ring that was green (for happy) and you'd feel happy? You can. Remember my earlier discussion about discarding clothing and saving only that which you feel great wearing? It is time to start thinking about this process in a grand way; it is time to start giving thought to simplifying your life and relationships. You may start with eliminating clothing that doesn't make you feel light and free; next you move to behaviors that do not work for you anymore; eventually you are going to come to limiting or eliminating altogether relationships that are toxic or damaging.

For today, it is enough to know that this is ahead of you and to begin to give thought to both the letting go and the receiving that will be a part of your conscious future.

■ **A CONSCIOUS LIVING PRACTICE FOR TODAY** ■

Below, think about one material change and one behavioral change that you have made since beginning your journey. Then think about one relational change that is ahead of you.

1. Material: _____.
2. Behavioral: _____.
3. Relational: _____.

....

AUGUST 20

To lose is to learn.—ANONYMOUS

SHIFTING PERCEPTION

One of the beauties of the complex human mind is its ability to shift perceptions quickly. To illustrate this point, think of a glass of water filled to the halfway mark. You may think of it as half-empty or half-full, yet you can also shift to the exact opposite perception in the blink of an eye.

Then consider another shift in perception. If you are seeing the glass through the "eyes of the mind," you use the powers of the mind to make a judgment of whether the glass is half-empty or half-full. If you made a shift to seeing through the "eyes of the heart," you might simply feel grateful for the existence of water and a glass in which to carry it. You wouldn't worry about whether it was empty or full . . . you would appreciate it as it is, for the gift of its existence.

■ A CONSCIOUS LIVING PRACTICE FOR TODAY ■

Today, experiment with seeing through the eyes of the heart. Whenever you notice yourself judging, evaluating, or comparing things—seeing through the eyes of the mind—shift to appreciating them as they are.

If you're strong enough, there are no precedents.—F. SCOTT FITZGERALD

THE ARTIST WITHIN

Everyone has an artist in their heart. Perhaps the artist shows his or her spirit in a visual art—painting, writing, photography—or maybe in another form, such as cooking, child-rearing, or teaching. The possibilities are endless. What are you doing to indulge your artist within, to give voice to your creative self?

As you get older, many of you leave the artist behind, usually standing lonely beside the once-playful, lighthearted child that you were. As you rush off to work or a Little League game or the market, you protest that there is no time for that kind of nonsense anymore. After all, your artist-self is hardly helping to pay the mortgage.

If your artist within is starving, then your spirit is starving. You cannot cut off a true part of yourself—and everyone has an artist in his or her heart—without doing damage to the rest of who you are. Spend a few moments remembering how you used to create, and commit yourself to carving out the time in your busy adult life for continued creation.

■ A CONSCIOUS LIVING PRACTICE FOR TODAY ■

When you were younger, what dreams did you have that involved creating? What were you going to be when you grew up? What was the career that no longer made sense as you got older and realized you had to earn a living?

Welcome your artist back into your life. Commit yourself to fifteen minutes of fame for your artist-within during the next twenty-four hours. Write it—in pen—in your daybook. Keep the agreement with yourself. Draw, doodle, write, dance, sing, play an instrument, bake, juggle, or close your eyes and allow yourself a fifteen-minute fantasy in which you're a famous actor, director, composer . . . give yourself the gift of allowing your creative self to awaken again. Pay attention to how you feel as your artist awakens, and to the ways in which the awakening carries forth into the rest of your day.

....

AUGUST 22

His life was gentle, and the elements
So mixed in him that nature might stand up
And say to all the world, "This was a man!"—WILLIAM SHAKESPEARE

SMALL ACTS OF KINDNESS

One of the profound discoveries of relationship psychology, derived from hundreds of studies, surveys, and interviews, is ... (drum roll, please!) ... people in thriving relationships are nicer to each other. What the concept of niceness translates to in action terms is that they perform small acts of kindness for each other.

In thriving relationships, people do kind things for each other on a regular basis. I was once in a group of perhaps a dozen people at a conference. There was a couple in their sixties to my right. I heard the man lean over and ask his wife, "Could I get you a cup of tea?" She smiled and nodded. I watched him go over to the beverage area and make her tea. The care he put into it was worthy of any Japanese tea ceremony. He brought it back and carefully handed it to her, and she received the gift with a quick kiss on his cheek. I suddenly found tears coming out of my eyes at the sacredness of this small interaction.

■ A CONSCIOUS LIVING PRACTICE FOR TODAY ■

As you move through your day, look for opportunities to carry out small acts of kindness. Whether with strangers or people you know, be vigilant for things you could do that would make their moment with you better.

AUGUST 23

The work of the individual still remains the spark that moves mankind forward.
—IGOR SIKORSKY

THE KING OF THE WORLD

If you saw *Titanic* (and if you didn't, you're one of a handful), you'll remember a scene in which the male lead, a materially poor young man, stands at the tip of the bow holding on to a railing, his body out over the water, his arms spread wide as the majestic ship cuts through the ocean. "I'm the king of the world!" he cries out gleefully from his perch above it all.

There may be few times when you feel that sweeping, giddy sense of ownership of the world. Disappointments happen, events go spinning out of your hands, the world does not treat you with the respect or gentleness for which you might hope. It is your choice how you handle the realities, large and small, that color your existence. Are you bowed down by reality, or do you use it as a springboard from which you can proclaim your strength in the face of disaster, your hardiness in the face of cutting winds and stinging saltwater?

You are the king—or the queen—of the world: of *your* world. The only question is whether you recognize this. You are the central figure in the drama that is your life. What is it going to be? A tragedy? A comedy of errors? A bittersweet love story? Or a little of everything, a play in which you are a participant, not just an observer, and a performance that leaves you satisfied when the curtain closes?

■ A CONSCIOUS LIVING PRACTICE FOR TODAY ■

Imagine for a moment that your life is, indeed, a film. How would you classify it? Is it a comedy, a tragedy, or something else altogether? Now think about what you'd like for your life to be. If people reviewed it, what would you want them to say? Use the "thought starts" below to help you.

My life as film is best described as a _____.

The story of my life can be reviewed as being _____.

....

AUGUST 24

The strength of a nation derives from the integrity of the home.—CONFUCIUS

THE COMFORTS OF HOME

We often love—and cling to—that which is familiar. In studies of victims of child abuse, it is proved, time and again, that children view their abusive parents with something akin to worship and long to return to the abusing or neglectful parent even when living in a far more loving alternative home. This is, in part, due to the belief the child develops that he or she is responsible for the abuse; returning to it offers the opportunity to "get it right," in a sense. In part, too, the clinging to that which is negative and harmful is related to your comfort with the familiar; no matter how destructive, the familiar is what you know, and therefore, you cling to it like a lifeboat.

Each of you clings to something, or to many things, that have long since stopped providing you succor. Material objects, jobs, people . . . you hold on for dear life even when you are being battered, whether the battering is physical or emotional. On a conscious journey, the familiar unworkable, which I have already discussed, begins to lose its appeal, and as this occurs, you are given the opportunity to let it fall away from you. In this opportunity, however, you are also given the choice of clinging even more desperately to that which harms you. What will it be? The familiar or the new? The hope or the despair? Becoming conscious means breathing deeply, and sometimes it means sucking in a huge gasp of air and then leaping into the unknown. Make the leap.

■ A CONSCIOUS LIVING PRACTICE FOR TODAY ■

Identify something you have let go of in your life. Consider the material, behavioral, or relational change you have made. Breathe deeply, centering yourself as you close your eyes for a moment and celebrate your courage in letting go of something that once seemed essential.

....

AUGUST 25

A man's dying is more the survivors' affair than his own.—THOMAS MANN

MERCY AND GRACE

Laura writes: On the day of my grandfather's funeral, I stood in front of the church. The limousine that carried my mother, her three sisters, and her brother was only a few feet away. As I talked to an old family friend, we were both distracted by noises coming from the limousine. Looking at it, we became aware that it was actually shaking slightly, and from inside, despite its closed windows and doors, we could both hear what sounded like wailing.

"Those poor kids," sympathized the friend, shaking his head as he imagined the grief-torn family inside the limo. "They're completely torn up. They're crying so hard they're actually shaking the car."

I nodded solemnly, but something struck me as odd. I'd heard those sounds before in my raucous family, and they weren't wailing sounds. Sure enough, when I pulled my mother aside at the small luncheon later, she surreptitiously looked around and then grinned. She said:

"We were telling funny stories about Daddy and laughing. What you heard was wailing, yes, but we were wailing with laughter." I must have looked at her somewhat askance. "You think Grandpa wouldn't have been right in there with us, egging us on?" she asked. And she was right.

I have learned both love and loss at my mother's knee, and this is perhaps the most important lesson I have learned: laughter soothes; laughter heals. In everything, there is a space, waiting to be filled, for laughter.

■ A CONSCIOUS LIVING PRACTICE FOR TODAY ■

There are two ways to view a red nose: it can be the result of tears, or it can be a clown's nose, pointing out absurdity, humor, silliness. Think back on a time of grief and a moment when you, perhaps, found something humorous in the grief. Did you censor yourself or did you allow yourself the acceptance to be healed with humor?

....

AUGUST 26

For the unlearned, old age is winter;
for the learned, it is the season of the harvest.—HASIDIC PROVERB

WHEN I AM A YOUNG WOMAN, I SHALL . . .

Laura writes: Not long ago I read a lovely collection of poetry, essays, and art. The book, *When I Am an Old Woman, I Shall Wear Purple*, celebrates aging with exuberance, spontaneity, and individuality. Must you wait until the children are raised, the retirement is achieved, and the bones in your body protest before you feel free to make contact with that which is most unique, most free, most *you* about you? Why waste so many years in a staid, predictable, don't-rock-the-boat mentality? It is true that your children may bow their heads with embarrassment at the sight of you spontaneously dancing in the park, but, I assure you, if your children are above the age of ten and under the age of thirty or so, they will bow their heads in embarrassment regardless of what you do. So your colleagues, your family members, will look at you as if you've lost your mind when you sing loudly in the elevator, when you tell a truth that has been banging around inside your careful head, when you cry openly at something that moves you. My response and theory is, perhaps, not phrased in quite the way that a textbook on human behavior and psychology might phrase it, but despite that, my response is . . . so what? *So what?* And so I began wearing hats. It hardly qualifies as radical, and yet, despite loving hats, I had avoided them because I worried that people might look at me oddly.

I, in my fiftieth year, started writing a screenplay, despite the insistence of some that I should stick to what I know best and have achieved success at—nonfiction relationship/personal growth books—in order to avoid the possibility of failure.

What aren't you doing because of your fear?

■ A CONSCIOUS LIVING PRACTICE FOR TODAY ■

Identify one thing you'd love to do—wear a hat, write a poem, sing at an open-mike night at a local pub—and then . . . do it.

....

AUGUST 27

It proves, on close examination, that work is less boring than amusing oneself.
—CHARLES BAUDELAIRE

COLD TURKEY

I have already spent some time discussing the narcotics that are used to numb the pain and the joy of human existence. Today, more than two-thirds of the way into this year of journey, I ask you to focus on television and its place in your life. Some people do not own televisions by choice, and others do not have televisions by circumstance, but most people—even the very poorest, even those in the most remote areas of the world, living without indoor plumbing—not only own televisions but have set up those televisions as guests of honor throughout the house. The sets occupy eye-drawing positions, resting on precious pieces of furniture, adorned with all sorts of accoutrements: remote-control devices so that only wrist movement is necessary, VCRs, cable boxes to allow access to hundreds of options for zoning out. More than drugs, more than alcohol, televisions have become the narcotic of choice in our culture. This is not to suggest that television is not a remarkable medium, one that can bring vital information, connection to people and places that were once beyond us. Television is both of these things and much more. And yet, it is also the most prevalent way in which people flee, avoid, deny, and escape reality and relationship. You watch the suffering on a soap opera, and yet cannot see the suffering in your own home. You gasp at the danger in a thriller, and yet cannot see the crisis in your partner's eyes.

If each time you approached the television, you first asked yourself what else you could be doing, with whom you could be engaging, what might the answer be?

■ A CONSCIOUS LIVING PRACTICE FOR TODAY ■

For the next twenty-four hours, your television is broken. Commit yourself to doing anything but watching television. Feel what you feel as you do this; you may find yourself feeling cut adrift, or you may feel a sense of despair—we often do when we give up our crutches—and this is all right. Let yourself feel whatever arises, and do not judge yourself, but do not give in to the feelings by "medicating" yourself with the television. Read, talk, watch your loved ones, walk, dream, write, or sit with your eyes open and do absolutely nothing at all. Just be.

AUGUST 28

Doubt is not a pleasant condition, but certainty is.—Voltaire

THAT WHICH IS REAL

Who are you most sure of in your life? What is trust—and can you trust it? Today your work is to look at your relationships under the gentle—but bright—light of the truth. Who is most central to you, and to whom are you most central? Are they the same people? What most defines these central relationships in which you are involved? If trust, truth, and acceptance are not the defining features of these relationships, it is time to begin rethinking and redrawing them. You have the ability—and the absolute right—to do so.

■ A CONSCIOUS LIVING PRACTICE FOR TODAY ■

Think of two or three of the most significant relationships in your life. Think of the dominant emotional tone of each relationship: joy, fear, love, despair. Then, zoom in to a closer focus: What is missing in each of these relationships? Sometimes what's missing is laughter; other times it's accountability. Only you know what's missing, and until you do, it will be difficult to find out if the missing element can be found.

....

AUGUST 29

Where we love is home—home that our feet may leave but not our hearts.
—Oliver Wendell Holmes

SECURITY BLANKETS

Laura writes: It occurred to me that my three sons have never had security blankets, or any type of object of affection of that nature. Many children carry around an old, torn blanket, or a pacifier, or a stuffed animal that is coming apart at the seams; the object is familiar, loved, and necessary to the child's sense of safety and ownership in the world. I immediately worried—as parents will—about whether my sons' lack of security objects said something about their ability to form close attachments. Looking around, though, I reassured myself; they are deeply attached to me, to their father, and to each other, and they each have strong preferences in food, clothing, play.

It occurred to me that my sons carry their sense of safety and security within, and this, more than anything, reassured me. It is what I wish for you, that your safety, and a sense of your sanctity, become internalized, interior, so that as you encounter the unfamiliar, as you journey on paths that you have not yet taken, you are accompanied by a guide who lives within you, one who steers you unerringly in the direction in which you need to go—not always the *easy* way, but the *right* way for you—and one who blankets you in a warm, loving embrace along the path.

■ A CONSCIOUS LIVING PRACTICE FOR TODAY ■

Think of an object of affection—a security blanket, if you will—that you currently have in your life. Perhaps it is a piece of jewelry, or maybe something far larger, such as your home. Consider what the object represents to you: security, safety, constancy, your personal history, and so on. How can you transfer these feelings into your essence, into your interior life? I am not suggesting that you rid yourself of the object of affection, but that you identify ways in which to transfer the associated positive feelings inside of your heart to be carried with you wherever you go and whatever you do.

Everything that is done in the world is done by hope.—MARTIN LUTHER

THE PRACTICE OF CONFESSION

You have probably heard of (or perhaps experienced) the Catholic practice of confession, in which you share your sins with a priest, ask for forgiveness, and then perform an act of penance to make up for the sins. You mirror this practice in everyday life if you are in conscious relationship. You open yourself to awareness of the mistakes you make and commit to honesty with others about those mistakes, and then you try to make things right.

To admit to a mistake—large or small—is a fearful business for many people. The worry seems to be that admitting to a mistake will make you less of a person; it will acknowledge your imperfections to a wider audience. And, in fact, it does broadcast your imperfections, but this is a good thing. By admitting to your humanity—the imperfection that lives in you—you become more fully human, and more fully connected with others, who know that they, too, are imperfect.

■ A CONSCIOUS LIVING PRACTICE FOR TODAY ■

Imagine yourself as both confessor and confessee—in other words, you are both priest and parishioner to yourself. What might you admit about yourself? What have you done lately that is not in keeping with your integrity? Focus on one thing you have done that points to your imperfection, and then spend a moment loving yourself for both your imperfection and your honesty in knowing about your imperfection. And now make it right: identify a way in which you can acknowledge and expiate this behavior. Almost always, expiation comes when you expose your imperfections to the accepting light of day.

AUGUST 31

Not everything that is faced can be changed. But nothing can be changed until it is faced.
—JAMES BALDWIN

THE CORRECT POSITION FOR A TOILET SEAT

Does the toilet seat lid belong up or down when not in use? I once had a client insist that if God had intended for toilets to remain open, he would not have made them with lids. I question whether there is a god involved in the manufacture of toilets, but the real point, of course, is insisting that you have the insider track on how reality is supposed to be. Squeeze or roll toothpaste tubes? Stop and ask directions, or blunder along and perhaps see a beautiful sight along the way? Toilet seats up or down? The questions are endless, and the questions are small, insignificant, unless you consider them in the context of compromise: how much must I compromise in order to be in a successful relationship?

■ A CONSCIOUS LIVING PRACTICE FOR TODAY ■

Identify an ongoing, small (some might say petty) conflict between you and your partner, or a past partner if you are not currently in a partner relationship. Consider the extent to which you are clinging to your position. The harder you cling, the less likely it is that your position has anything to do with the actual issue. Instead, your insistence is related to your need to control, to your need to be right. Take several deep breaths and repeat the following affirmation: *I do not need to be right. I am good even when I am not right.*

And now, let go of the conflict. Then identify how you are going to compromise. This is about you, not about your partner. It is irrelevant what your partner does; what you do is essential, and of your essence.

• The conflict: _____.
• The compromise: _____.

SEPTEMBER

A good indignation brings out all one's powers.—RALPH WALDO EMERSON

REFRAMING ANGER

Laura writes: I was living at home during college and walked in on an argument between my mother and stepfather. I was instantly filled with deep anxiety. In my distant personal history, I had the misfortune of hearing *only one argument* between my mother and father. That had occurred on the evening before they announced that they were getting divorced, and although I knew *intellectually* that anger and loss weren't necessarily connected, the two were still deeply intertwined for me. On this occasion, both my mother and my stepdad were obviously furious, and they sounded like fishwives, their voices high-pitched and shrieking. Stomping down the hall, my stepfather left the house, slamming the door on his way out. My anxiety was just shooting up through the roof when he came back.

"Honey?" he said, in a sorrowful and apologetic tone. I breathed a sigh of relief; everything was going to be fine. He was going to back down or apologize.

"Yes?" my mother answered sweetly, obviously also sure that he was prepared to apologize.

Suddenly, he raised his hand and gave her the finger, a huge grin on his face.

I cringed, my eyes closed, waiting in that long moment's silence; surely she was going to order him away forever. What I heard next changed my life.

Laughter. They both erupted suddenly into laughter. They both intuitively knew that they had been rigid, unfair, and unpleasant, and *they were good enough friends, with big enough hearts, and small enough egos,* to find a way to say so to each other and move on.

You sometimes regress to a child's position when you are most angry. You may call names, silently or aloud, or you may cling to your position as if it is a precious toy that you cannot stand to share. Next time you are in anger, allow yourself to see a way—or ways—in which you are childlike. Then encourage yourself to be open enough, expansive enough, loving enough, to love the child within you.

- My childlike behavior: _____.
- What's in it for me: _____.

....

SEPTEMBER 2

All the wonders you seek are within yourself.—SIR THOMAS BROWN

MIND/BODY/SPIRIT: AN ESSENTIAL UNITY

The fields of psychology and medicine have begun to take seriously what common sense has whispered in our ears for thousands of years: Body, mind, and spirit are linked in one whole we call ourselves. After much experience—with my own illnesses as well as with my clients—I have come to believe that the majority of our physical ills have their origin in emotional and spiritual issues we have not dealt with successfully. When your mind is confused, when your heart is heavy, when your soul is divided, you are ripe for illness to get a grip on you.

The next time you feel sick, pay close attention to all aspects of yourself. Certainly take your medicine and follow good medical advice, but also listen to the messages from your heart and soul. The last time I had a sore throat, a friend of mine performed an instant cure by asking me one question over the phone. It was: What are you afraid to say? I reflected on it for a few moments, then told him about something I'd been afraid to talk to my wife about. I wanted to change some travel plans but hadn't told her because I was afraid she'd get upset. As soon as I said it my throat began to clear. Then I went in the living room, took a deep breath, and told her. She had a momentary flash of irritation, but it soon melted and she felt fine about it. My throat had been speaking loudly, but through the medium of pain, and when I allowed my voice box to do the speaking, the pain disappeared.

■ A CONSCIOUS LIVING PRACTICE FOR TODAY ■

Take a moment to float an affirmation through your mind: *I pay attention to my body, mind, and spirit, and I listen carefully to messages from all of myself.*

....

SEPTEMBER 3
Sex is an emotion in motion.——MAE WEST

LOVE AND LUST

It is not at all unusual to go through a phase of sexual exploration in life, when you may have a number of different sexual partners and engage in a wide range of sexual behaviors. For many people, this exploration coincides with the first period of freedom—the college years, or the first apartment, or, for some, after a divorce. It is, of course, no secret that having a number of sexual partners is potentially deadly these days. What about the effects, though, on your heart?

I've seen the following visual example used: take two pieces of masking tape and stick them together. They stick well the first time. Take them apart and restick them. A little less sticky this time. The more often you bond the two pieces together and take them apart, the less ability each has to bond. Indiscriminate sexuality with multiple partners not only poses huge health risks, it creates the potential for damage to your ability to bond with another. I stress the distinction of *indiscriminate* sexuality here; I am not talking about sexual intimacy within the context of a loving, mutual, and respectful relationship.

For the next several days I will discuss conscious sexuality. I will help you to identify the place that sexuality has in your life: who you are as a sexual being, what values you have that are related to sexuality and intimacy, and how you can reach a comfortable place that honors your values and treats your sexual self with respect, joy, passion, and purpose.

■ A CONSCIOUS LIVING PRACTICE FOR TODAY ■

Think back on the messages you received about sexuality as a child. Did your family treat the subject with openness or embarrassment? Did you ever see your parents touching or behaving sexually? When you touched yourself as a child, what was the response from your parents? Think on these questions and on how your sexual upbringing is with you still today. (No changes for today; for now you are just getting reacquainted with the beginnings of your sexual self.)

....

SEPTEMBER 4

Lord, make me chaste—but not yet.—St. Augustine

THE CONSCIOUS SEXUAL SELF

Do you know who you are sexually? Are you conscious of what brings you the most pleasure and what makes you most uncomfortable—and why—and how sexuality can both nurture and make use of your creativity?

I believe that conscious sexuality is about both *passion* and *purpose*. In the conscious sexual life, you nourish and give a voice to the sexual being that has grown out of the merging of your physical and emotional selves. In conscious sexuality, you also honor your emotional and physical integrity by treating your sexuality with both open, honest joyfulness and a well-tempered sense of responsibility.

I've noticed that the sexiest people I know seem to be that way because they are truly alive and truly engaged with the world around them. They are full of excitement as they live creatively and purposefully and with commitment to their world. This engagement with the world shows in their glowing eyes, their proud carriage, their graceful walk.

I believe that carrying on a love affair with life makes one most open to the deepest of love affairs with another.

■ A CONSCIOUS LIVING PRACTICE FOR TODAY ■

Identify a situation that is not traditionally sexy, but when you have felt most sexual. Perhaps you were working out, or dancing alone, or teaching someone and seeing the understanding dawn in your student's eyes. Perhaps you were hammering a nail into the walls that would become a new home for a family in need, or perhaps you were creating art. What about this time makes it come to mind now?

- I was at my most sexual when I was _____.
- I was (emotionally) feeling _____.
- I was (physically) feeling _____.
- I could recreate this sense for myself by _____.

What is life, what is joy without golden Aphrodite?
May I die when these things no longer move me:
hidden love affairs, sweet nothings and bed.—MIMNERMUS

SEXUAL VALUES AND THE VALUE OF SEX

Over the course of your life, the value you assign to sex, and the values that you relate to sex, can change. An example of the value you assign to sex: research shows that the typical teenage boy, for instance, thinks about sex every eight seconds. The adult who tries that is going to be mightily distracted from pressing issues such as work and family. As to values: a younger person might be more focused on the importance of "getting some" while an older person might be more focused on a merging of physical and emotional intimacy with his or her partner and the gestalt of sex: the means rather than the end.

It is essential, if you are to have a conscious sexuality, that you know yourself and that you be true to that knowledge of who you are and what you value, sexually and otherwise. In all areas, you often enter adulthood wearing the mantle of your parents' values, and while these values *may* work well for you, I believe it is essential that you arrive at your values after due consideration of what *you* want in your life.

This is conscious living: listening carefully for your own voice and then letting that voice sing out, whether the song is about your creativity, your intellectual self, your sexuality, your social self, or your physical self.

■ A CONSCIOUS LIVING PRACTICE FOR TODAY ■

A value is a belief to live by, something you practice rather than something you just preach. What are your values when it comes to sexuality and sexual practices? Use the thought starters below to help you as you think about your values and your sexuality:

- When it comes to sex, I believe that _____.
- I would not be comfortable with _____.
- A good sexual relationship requires _____.

....

How could the drops of water know themselves to be a river?
Yet the river flows on.——ANTOINE DE SAINT-EXUPÉRY

FINDING SAFETY THROUGH RESONANCE

The first lesson of conscious living invites you to resonate with life, and to feel your way through to the larger space of your whole self. Think of yourself for a moment as a beautiful acoustic guitar. Life is always playing your strings, and sometimes none too gently. If you try to arrange it so that life doesn't get to you—so that your strings are never plucked—you don't get to hear the music. If you let your strings go slack, through disuse or lack of care, you never get to know what you could sound like. If you keep yourself in tune, you can hear all the overtones and *vibrations* of yourself and your neighboring strings. It is the space within the guitar that makes the sound what it is. If you become sensitive, you can hear the silent space at the heart and soul of your instrument, the very source from which all sound emerges.

■ A CONSCIOUS LIVING PRACTICE FOR TODAY ■

Put on a piece of instrumental music that you're fond of. Close your eyes and listen to the instruments, listening for which one most calls out to you. Visualize yourself as that instrument, and imagine the care that must go into keeping your notes strong and clear and beautiful. Don't hurry or rush this exercise; take your time as you let the music fill you with the sound of essence.

My great mistake, the fault for which I can't forgive myself, is that one day I ceased my obstinate pursuit of my own individuality.—OSCAR WILDE

THE POWER OF ESSENCE

There is a great deal of power in accessing the space of pure consciousness within yourself. Once you feel it you can never have any more doubts about the divine nature of the universe and your connection to it. The space you feel in your body and mind feels seamlessly connected to the space at large in the cosmos. The space feels organically divine, as the drinking of water feels organically thirst-quenching compared to seeing the formula for water on a chalkboard. The Zen writer D. T. Suzuki called it the "lightning-and-thunder discovery that the universe and oneself *are not* remote and apart, but an intimate, palpitating whole."

The Native American visionary Black Elk spoke his version of this principle in this way: "The first peace, which is the most important, is that which comes in the souls of people when they realize their relationship, their oneness, with the universe and all its powers, and when they realize at the center of the universe dwells the Great Spirit, and that the center is really everywhere. It is within each one of us."

■ A CONSCIOUS LIVING PRACTICE FOR TODAY ■

Think on what Spirit means to you. Is it a force outside of yourself? A powerful peace within? How can you merge the external experiencing of Spirit with the internal living of peace and wholeness?

SEPTEMBER 8

A man cannot be comfortable without his own approval.—MARK TWAIN

TAKING RESPONSIBILITY FOR YOUR FEELINGS

People make a great leap forward in well-being and productivity when they claim responsibility for their feelings. Many leaders in the fields of psychiatry and psychology consider that to be the crucial move that creates success and happiness. Until you claim full responsibility for your feelings, there is always a tendency to believe your feelings are caused by other people, a perception that puts you in the victim position.

Logically, it is unarguable that you are the source of your feelings. If you, John Gotti, and the Dalai Lama are all in a 7–11 when a robber comes in to hold up the store, you might feel scared, the Dalai Lama might feel compassion, and Gotti might break the robber's kneecaps. Each of you would source a completely different emotional response to the same event.

■ A CONSCIOUS LIVING PRACTICE FOR TODAY ■

Repeat each sentence in your mind, giving accent to the first word in the sentence. After each repetition, pause for five to ten seconds to notice any response your mind has to the sentence.

I cause my anger.
I cause my hurt feelings.
I cause my fears.
I cause my excitement.
I cause my happiness.

What are you pretending not to know?
—Graffiti discovered in Harvard Business School lounge

THE OSTRICH MANEUVER

It takes energy—genuine physical energy—to avoid knowing things that you need to learn. Another way to say this is that you organize learning experiences for yourself, then refuse to get the lesson until it's administered by sledgehammer. Then you often say, "Why me?" This is the way of the ostrich, who deals with overstimulation by sticking its head into the ground. Trouble is, this maneuver exposes vulnerable parts of yourself to the breeze. There is only one way out of this dilemma, and that's to make an openhearted and open-minded commitment to learning what you most need to learn. When you make a full-scale commitment to learning from every interaction, life smooths out marvelously.

■ A CONSCIOUS LIVING PRACTICE FOR TODAY ■

Say this sentence aloud and in your mind a few times, until you can feel it in your body: *I commit to learning and growing from every interaction I have today.*

....

SEPTEMBER 10

Few is the number who think with their own minds and feel with their own hearts.
—Albert Einstein

THE LOST ART OF THINKING FOR YOURSELF

I once heard a stunning sermon by a minister named Wallace Hamilton, who was speaking at a statewide church gathering. Although this was in the conservative and conforming South of the early sixties,

Dr. Hamilton's message was radical and electrifying. He told us to think for ourselves, to feel what was true in our own hearts. He cautioned us to beware of those who would sell us a comfortable prison called security. He urged us not to fall into the trance of consumerism, ending up with a house full of appliances and a heart empty of value. I was deeply moved not only by the content of his remarks but by his courage in delivering them in the climate of the times. The journey of conscious living is a path of constant inquiry into what is true and what is real. It is not a path of constant vigilance for what is popular and acceptable. Ultimately, it is a path that takes you, step by step, beyond what is even thought possible.

■ A CONSCIOUS LIVING PRACTICE FOR TODAY ■

As you go through your day, notice your thoughts and feelings. Ask yourself, "Where did these thoughts come from? Where did these feelings come from? Are these my authentic thoughts and feelings, or did someone else program me to think them?" In very practical terms, is that cheeseburger you're hungry for an authentic desire of your body, or is it the result of last night's TV commercial?

SEPTEMBER 11
Believe one who has tried it.—VIRGIL

SALUTING A PAST MASTER

Epictetus was a well-known teacher of conscious living who worked in Rome during a time of great upheaval. Born into slavery, he had risen by the penetrating power of his teachings. Then, a wave of fundamentalism swept through, spearheaded by the zeal of the early Christians. Teachers such as Epictetus were run out of Rome and had to take up residence in faraway places. People continued to seek out Epictetus, though, and fortunately one of his students wrote down the essence of his teachings. If you go to a twelve-step meeting anywhere in the world, you'll make Epictetus's acquaintance in a most practical form: The Serenity Prayer, recited every day by millions of sincere people, is based on his teaching of two thousand years ago. Few people today have even heard the name of the emperor Domitian, who had the bad taste to run Epictetus out of town.

■ A CONSCIOUS LIVING PRACTICE FOR TODAY ■

In honor of Epictetus, ask yourself: What do I know that could help people change their lives two thousand years from now? What do I believe in that would be worth running me out of town for? What do I know that would make people come from far away to learn, even after I'd been run out of town?

....

SEPTEMBER 12

I always prefer to believe the best of everybody—it saves so much trouble.
—RUDYARD KIPLING

PRE-PAVING WITH APPRECIATION

Even a small amount of appreciation (if sincere) can create a wave of positive energy throughout the day. One of my friends has a technique he calls pre-paving, which uses the power of appreciation to enhance interactions with people. Here's how it works: In bed, before the day begins, he generates appreciations for key people he's likely to see that day. He focuses particular attention on people with whom he has difficult relationships. His goal is to send a wave of positive energy through the potential sticky places in his relationship with them. He makes extravagant claims for the benefits of pre-paving, and my experience with the technique supports his enthusiasm. Give it a try, and see if it works for you.

■ A CONSCIOUS LIVING PRACTICE FOR TODAY ■

Pause for a minute to think through some of the interactions you're likely to have today. Think of some of the people you'll connect with, remembering to include some of those with whom you have difficult relationships. As you bring them to mind, imagine beaming a wave of appreciation at them. Feel a moment of genuine appreciation for each of them.

....

SEPTEMBER 13

How often we find ourselves turning our backs on our actual friends, that we might go and meet their ideal cousins.—HENRY DAVID THOREAU

THE ART OF ORGANIC FORGIVENESS

Forgiveness is a subtle art that has huge benefits. One of the reasons it is not more widely practiced is that we don't preface our forgiveness with acceptance. Many well-intentioned people try to jump over their negative feelings to achieve forgiveness. Perhaps some people can seal off their negative feelings with a shift to forgiveness, but most of us find that unless we achieve an organic forgiveness, the negative feelings keep coming back.

The art of organic forgiveness rests on fully acknowledging your negative feelings for the person you're trying to forgive. When you can celebrate your anger or sadness about the person, you can often feel the blossoming of a more permanent form of forgiveness. The negative feelings you may have about the other person usually recede and disappear only after they are fully acknowledged.

■ A CONSCIOUS LIVING PRACTICE FOR TODAY ■

Today, do an experiment in organic forgiveness. Think of someone with whom you've had a troubled relationship. Instead of forcing yourself into an artificial feeling of forgiveness, thoroughly acknowledge your anger or sadness or betrayal or any other emotions you feel toward that person. Take a few breaths around those feelings, then open to forgiveness.

....

SEPTEMBER 14

I got the sun in the mornin' and the moon at night.—IRVING BERLIN

THE APPRECIATION OF ORDINARY THINGS

Most of you are familiar with one definition of appreciation, the one that means to speak positively of someone or something. There's another definition of appreciation, though, that's also worth knowing. It's to be "sensitively aware" of something, as a movie critic might appreciate the way a film is edited, while others might not give any thought to its editing at all.

Being sensitively aware of the ordinary and overlooked parts of life can have a powerful benefit. A woman of my acquaintance spent a weekend at a sensory awareness workshop, during which she was given the assignment of spending an hour eating one fresh cherry. The exercise made such an impact on her that she lost thirty pounds over the next few months by practicing mindful eating. With no change in her diet or activity level, she eliminated a weight problem with which she'd struggled for years. By refocusing on what her body needed and by being totally focused on the experience of meeting the needs of her body, she redefined her relationship with food.

Do a thirty-second experiment in appreciation right now. Look around your environment until your eye lights on something ordinary—something you may have seen a thousand times before. Go to it and study it carefully for thirty seconds. Appreciate it, in the sense of being sensitively aware of it. If you like, pause for this experiment several times throughout the day.

....

SEPTEMBER 15

I do not seek. I find.——PABLO PICASSO

THE ART OF ENJOYMENT

On the path of conscious living, one of your very highest priorities is to create peace of mind and body. If you can harmonize the being of human beings, everything you do is affected. Your moods have a profound effect on everything in life. You can prove this to yourself very easily. Notice that when your mood is high and harmonious, you see the world in a better light and you treat others better. When your mood drops, you begin to think negative thoughts and you see people in a more negative way.

One of my friends has a classic car over which he fusses endlessly. When he is in a high mood, he looks out at this car and sees a beautiful treasure that he is proud to own. When he is in a low mood, he sees the same car as an upkeep nightmare, a money drain, and a source of friction between him and his wife. The car never changes, but his view of it shifts with his mood. And that is true for each and every one of you. When you're in a high mood, the world is full of possibility. When you're in a low mood, the world looks unsafe and limited. You need to learn a great deal about your moods so you can have moods without them having you.

Make today a mood-awareness day. Simply study the fluctuation of your moods—notice when you're up and when you're down. Notice that the quality of your thoughts and your feelings will give you an instant barometer reading on your moods.

....

SEPTEMBER 16

All that we are arises with our thoughts.—BUDDHA

A NEW RELATIONSHIP WITH THOUGHT

Begin to cultivate a new relationship with your thoughts. Don't judge them or criticize them; just notice them. This is a powerful practice for several reasons. First, you can notice how your thoughts are a mirror reflection of your moods. Notice that when your mood drops, the quality of your thoughts drops also. As you watch your thoughts, you will also begin to see that you are much more than your thoughts. Your ability to witness your thoughts—watching them go by like clouds passing through the sky—will give you a remarkable clarity about yourself. You'll see that your thoughts are just thoughts, not necessarily anything to take seriously. Your point of view is just your point of view, not right, not wrong, just the way you see things. Realizing this, you begin to understand that your point of view does not need defending. As you let go of the need to defend your point of view, you feel much greater security and peace of mind.

■ A CONSCIOUS LIVING PRACTICE FOR TODAY ■

Throughout the day, pause occasionally to make a formal shift in your attitude toward your thoughts. Beginning now, let go of judging your thoughts. Just let them flow—they're going to anyway! Take the brakes off and enjoy the flow of your thoughts without any criticism or judgment whatsoever. Take a vacation from judging your thoughts.

....

SEPTEMBER 17

Knowledge of what is possible is the beginning of happiness.——GEORGE SANTAYANA

BECOMING A MOOD-SMITH

The student of conscious living is a keen student of moods. You need to know the major secret of staying in a high mood. You need to know what makes moods drop, so you can know what to do when yours does. Don't try to get your mood to stay the same all the time—moods are designed to fluctuate somewhat. Your job is to notice when your mood is dropping and take steps to rebalance before it starts affecting the quality of your day. The big mistake people make with their moods is trying to change them from outside. Advertising would like you to believe that satisfaction can be yours by lighting up the right cigarette, and that you can feel better by drinking the right brand of fizzy sugar water. But this is all a pack of lies. The main thing that causes your mood to drop is the moment you slip out of integrity. Do that and your mood drops like a rock.

■ A CONSCIOUS LIVING PRACTICE FOR TODAY ■

Sharpen your sensitivity today to your moods. Notice the effects of the foods you eat and beverages you drink on your moods. Notice the effects of ignoring key feelings such as fear, sadness, and anger. Notice the effects of withholding truths from other people. As you learn to spot what makes your moods shift, you can take preventive action to stay high and clear.

SEPTEMBER 18

Whatever the universal nature assigns to any man at any time is for the good of that man at that time.—MARCUS AURELIUS

MORE ON MOODS

Integrity comes from a word that means "wholeness," so slipping out of integrity really means slipping out of wholeness. Your mood is an incredibly sensitive barometer to your state of integrity: any time you slip out of feeling connected to yourself, other people, or the universe around you, your mood will drop.

The first thing that will cause your mood to drop is ignoring a feeling. When you fail to acknowledge a feeling, when you override it or tune it out, your mood will drop. Understand—you don't need to act on feelings most of the time. You do not have to do anything with most of your feelings—they will blow right through like a breeze or a gust of wind. What you need to do is say hello to them and feel them. It is the act of ignoring them that causes moods to drop.

■ A CONSCIOUS LIVING PRACTICE FOR TODAY ■

Right now, pause and tune in to your feelings. Use your nonjudgmental awareness to feel your sensations and feelings. Throughout your day, pause occasionally to take this kind of "feeling snapshot." If you feel yourself slipping into a lower mood, be sure to pause for a tune-in.

....

SEPTEMBER 19

I will show you fear in a handful of dust.—T. S. ELIOT

THE SCOPE OF YOUR FEELINGS

Several main feelings flow through your body on a regular basis, along with a host of minor ones. The most common feeling is fear. Fear is felt mostly in the front of the body, in the stomach and chest. Most people feel it as an antsy, slightly queasy sensation, but all of you have your unique variation of it. The second most common feeling is hurt or sadness. The third is anger. A fourth is sexual feelings and sensations. If you study your feelings carefully, you will notice that many of your other feelings are actually variations of one of these main ones. Irritation and aggravation are minor variations of anger, for example, while anxiety is a milder version of fear. To stay balanced, you need to become expert at recognizing feelings. Think of this skill as something just as important as learning the alphabet in elementary school.

■ A CONSCIOUS LIVING PRACTICE FOR TODAY ■

As your day proceeds, make a practice of scanning the main "feeling zones" of your body. Check the front of your body—chest and belly—for sadness and fear. Check your shoulders, neck, and upper back for the tension of anger. Remember, you don't always need to do something with your feelings, such as express them or act on them. But noticing them—simply feeling them—is a key to staying in balance.

....

SEPTEMBER 20

Being entirely honest with oneself is a good exercise.—SIGMUND FREUD

THE COST OF HIDING SIGNIFICANT FEELINGS

A significant truth can be large or small. Of course, you don't want to go around all day babbling every little thing that goes on inside you, but you do need to speak significant truths. I once felt angry at a close friend for what I perceived as a slight. He had failed to call me on my birthday, as was our custom, and I withheld it instead of telling him I was angry and hurt. Soon, I found myself thinking negative thoughts about him. Fortunately, I spotted what I was doing when my mood was turning bleaker and bleaker. When I finally noticed it, I traced backward in time and found the moment I had withheld the feeling. I took a deep breath and picked up the phone and told him how I was feeling. To my surprise he burst into tears. He was going through a crisis in his marriage—his wife had just told him she was involved with another man, and he had been wanting to call me but had been ashamed to tell me about this. His withheld feeling had caused him to forget my birthday, and I, in turn, had made up my own drama about it. What could have turned into a life-long saga was cleared up in ten minutes of communication. As a result, our friendship bond deepened.

■ A CONSCIOUS LIVING PRACTICE FOR TODAY ■

Think of any relationships that have cooled or soured over the past couple of years. Ask yourself if it's been because of withheld feelings. If so, consider unburdening yourself to the key person involved.

....

SEPTEMBER 21

What comes from the heart, goes to the heart.—SAMUEL TAYLOR COLERIDGE

THE TRUTH DILEMMA

Telling the truth is a controversial subject, but there is a way to make it simple. There are books that argue that you should always tell the truth in all circumstances. Other books argue that you should be wary of telling the truth lest you disrupt those around you. The example that is often used is extramarital affairs. Let's say a man has an affair that is over and done with. Does he need to tell his wife about it? Which of the following two positions do you feel most comfortable with? Yes, he should tell his wife, because to withhold the secret puts him out of integrity and destroys any possibility of the kind of transparency that allows close relationships to flourish. Or no, he shouldn't tell, because to do so might hurt his wife needlessly.

■ A CONSCIOUS LIVING PRACTICE FOR TODAY ■

Based on your response to the dilemma posed above, do a cost-benefit analysis of how it has affected your life. In other words, if you said, "Yes, he should tell her," reflect on the costs and benefits that taking this position has resulted in for you. Do the same if you said he shouldn't tell.

....

SEPTEMBER 22

The age of miracles is forever here.—THOMAS CARLYLE

MESSAGES IN THE AIR

A scientific study done some years ago tells a lot about self-esteem problems. The scientists put small, voice-activated tape recorders on preschool children, then analyzed the tapes at the end of the week. Negative messages accounted for about 85 percent of the communications the children received: "Don't do that, quit it, be still, you're going to get hurt if you don't _____."

Conscious living involves becoming sensitive to the messages coming in at you every day, as well as becoming sensitive to the messages you're putting out into the world. You're a lot more sensitive to those messages than you probably realize. Surgeons, for example, are learning to be careful of what they say during surgery, lest negative messages get into patients while anesthetized.

■ A CONSCIOUS LIVING PRACTICE FOR TODAY ■

As you move through your day, pay attention to the tone and content of the messages people give each other (and you). Pay close attention to the words coming from your mouth, also. Discover your ratio of positive to negative messages.

....

SEPTEMBER 23

Who do I think I am, anyway?—GRAFFITI ON A WALL IN NEW YORK

MAKING THE BIG DISTINCTION

If you look at childhood pictures, you'll usually see a lot more light and wonder on faces than you see on those same faces by high school. The main reason is that as you grow you buy into other people's perceptions of you. If you think of yourself when you were conceived, you were a tiny chemical explosion of possibility. But not too long after that explosion of possibility, you were immersed in other people's thoughts and feelings about you. Did they want you? Did they love you? Whether they did or didn't, it was still only their perception of you. This perception was based on finances, problems they were wrestling with, timing, and other factors. Chances are it had nothing to do with you personally. They would have felt the same about anybody.

Part of the journey of conscious living is to separate who you actually are from who everyone else thinks you are. This distinction plays a role in every moment of your life.

■ A CONSCIOUS LIVING PRACTICE FOR TODAY ■

Reflect on this question for a moment: Who am I apart from others' perceptions of me? As you go through your day, apply this question to the key people with whom you interact. Who would I be apart from what this person thinks of me?

I have called the principle, by which each slight variation, if useful, is preserved, by the term of Natural Selection.—CHARLES DARWIN

SEEING THROUGH THE SCRIPT

The moment you were conceived, and certainly the moment you were born, you joined a family and a story already in progress when you came on the scene. Everyone's dramas were fully in place before you got there. Chances are, you became part of their drama. Their reactions to you became part of the drama—whether comedy or tragedy—of their lives. Regardless of who you were and what you represented, you had to fit into those dramas for your own survival. Faced with the choice of fitting in or not surviving, you fit in. Even if you rebelled against it, you were still reacting to those dramas. In other words, until you wake up to the family script, most of you are busily repeating the script or rebelling against it.

■ A CONSCIOUS LIVING PRACTICE FOR TODAY ■

Ask yourself what your family script is. If your family's history were a drama, what would the title be? Would it be a tale of a fight for survival? A tale of opposing forces in conflict? A travel story?

Ask yourself what your role is in the drama. Are you the prodigal son or daughter? The golden girl or boy? The one for whom all was sacrificed? Reflect on how this role has shaped your life.

SEPTEMBER 25

We never touch but at points.—Ralph Waldo Emerson

MASTERING THE TWO DIMENSIONS OF RELATIONSHIP

When most people think of relationship, they think of the flow of connection and closeness. While it's an important part of relationships, being close is only part of the process. Intimacy also depends on learning to be autonomous. In other words, embedded in intimacy are two distinct urges: merger and individuation. Most of you have not been aware of or responded to the pull toward both these natural relationship pulsations. In fact, many people have learned to doubt their relationships if one partner wants to have separate time, interests, or friends. On the path of conscious living, it's important to discover your unique "relationship dance" and to make your relationships big enough to encompass the different needs for unity and individuation that occur between partners and over time.

■ A CONSCIOUS LIVING PRACTICE FOR TODAY ■

Reflect for a moment on the way you've lived your relationship life. Based on your history, have you given more attention to merger or individuation? If you were rating each on a ten-point scale, what would your merger score be and what would your individuation score be? What can you learn from this that would be useful to you now in your relationship journey?

SEPTEMBER 26

The secret of success is constancy to purpose.—Benjamin Disraeli

GETTING COMFORTABLE WITH SUCCEEDING

As you become more successful, you may come up against the fear of abandoning others if you expand to your full potential. A successful entertainer of my acquaintance held herself back for many years by thinking this way. She unconsciously felt that if she kept herself unhappy and unsuccessful she would not have to leave behind people who were her friends when she was poor and struggling. She went through a period of punishing herself severely as she rose to greater success. Even after becoming a superstar, she felt miserable. Her mind had come up with the following twisted equation: even though I'm now wealthy and famous, if I can be miserable inside I won't be abandoning my old friends. In other words, if I can fail to enjoy my success, they'll forgive me for being rich and famous. With "a little help from her friends," she was able to let go of this way of thinking by having some conscious conversations with her old friends in which she shared her fears and found they loved her for herself, regardless of her success.

■ A CONSCIOUS LIVING PRACTICE FOR TODAY ■

Look around you at the various indicators of your success (or lack thereof). Ask yourself if there are ways you hold yourself back for fear of leaving others behind. If so, ask yourself if you could deal with the fear some way other than holding yourself hostage.

Love consists in this, that two solitudes protect and touch and greet each other.
—RAINER MARIA RILKE

ONLY LOVE

Only unconditional love is strong enough and big enough to encompass all the negativity you soak up in your life. Love is such a powerful healer because it's big enough to contain its opposite—you can love yourself for not being able to love yourself! Some of you may have been fortunate enough to be loved unconditionally as children. Not all of you were, however. I have worked with people who were born into situations where there was little or no love, or even basic caretaking. One of my first clients was a woman who'd been born in a concentration camp, after being conceived through a rape. Although orphaned at birth and beset on all sides by unspeakable horrors, she somehow not only survived but came to feel such unconditional love for herself and others that she was an inspiration to behold. By taking what she'd been given, working with it, and coming to love it as a part of her wholeness, she transcended it magnificently.

■ A CONSCIOUS LIVING PRACTICE FOR TODAY ■

Right now, take a moment to feel love for yourself. No matter what you've done or thought or felt in the past, no matter how you feel right now, feel love for yourself. If you can't, love yourself as much as you can for not being able to love yourself. Give yourself as much love as you can right now. A good way to get the flow of love going is to think of someone you know for sure you love . . . and to love yourself just like that.

SEPTEMBER 28

Quarrels would not last long if the fault was only on one side.
—La Rochefoucauld

CREATING AN ARGUMENT-FREE ZONE

If you want to create arguments, speak arguable concepts. This will guarantee argument wherever you go. While there's nothing wrong with argument itself, I recommend saving your arguments for times you can do them consciously. In close relationships, I recommend saying things that can't be argued about to the people with whom you want to become more intimate. The most unarguable areas I've discovered are: body sensations such as tension; core feelings such as anger and sadness; facts, such as broken agreements; interpretations, and fantasies, such as imagining a past flame during sex; and familiar patterns, such as noticing a way of interacting that reminds you of family gatherings. Creativity and renewed intimacy flourish in relationships in which partners practice speaking the unarguable truth.

■ A CONSCIOUS LIVING PRACTICE FOR TODAY ■

As an experiment, make a commitment to speaking only unarguable truths today. Begin with simple things: instead of saying, "It's a beautiful day" (which is always arguable), say something unarguable like, "I'm enjoying the sunshine today." Instead of giving a compliment by saying, "You're having a good hair day," substitute an unarguable truth, "I like the way your hair looks today." You will convey the same essential information, but in a way that eliminates argument.

Integrity simply means a willingness not to violate one's identity.——ERICH FROMM

ANOTHER WAY OF LOOKING AT RESPONSIBILITY

Most people assume that responsibility in close relationships means assigning the fault or assuming the burden. I learned from my students and clients that power struggles start the moment either partner steps out of 100 percent responsibility. For example, the most common complaints I've heard are "I'm tired of doing more than my share" and "I can't seem to get my partner to take more responsibility (or interest)." These complaints end only when each person chooses to take full, healthy responsibility for creating the issue or conflict. The heart of responsibility is genuine wondering, which is a whole-body experience not just a cognitive task. If my complainer stepped into 100 percent responsibility, he or she might say, "I wonder how and why I keep creating struggle in our relationship? I wonder how I could create genuine celebration in the daily household chores?" As people wonder, organic body wisdom has a chance to emerge and shift issues into creative solutions.

■ A CONSCIOUS LIVING PRACTICE FOR TODAY ■

Do a thirty-second experiment in body awareness: feel any places where you carry a sense of burden in your body. Feel any places where you carry a sense of blame or fault. When you can feel those places, replace the burden and blame with a sense of wondering. Feel wonder in those places . . . and introduce wonder to your body throughout the day.

The only people for me are the mad ones, the ones who are mad to live, mad to talk, mad to be saved . . . the ones who never yawn and say a commonplace thing, but burn, burn, burn like fabulous yellow roman candles exploding like spiders across the stars.
—JACK KEROUAC

PERSONAL ESSENCE AND UNIVERSAL ESSENCE

Your own essence has a personal flavor to it that makes it different from anybody else's essence. You can also feel a type of essence that goes beyond you, the feeling of connection with all things. To feel this universal essence, focus on the way we are all the same at the deepest level. Ultimately, your self-esteem is rooted in feeling your essence and the essence of all beings. As your awareness grows, you begin to realize that who you really are is untouched by any message you've received or any life experience you've had. There is a part of you that has always been exactly the same, completely free and untouched by any of life's events.

■ A CONSCIOUS LIVING PRACTICE FOR TODAY ■

Pause to feel your personal essence right this moment. Feel in your body and mind the way you've always been the same since you can remember . . . the feeling inside that's remained steady since forever. That's your essence, your essential self. Life can be up or down, high or low, rough or smooth, and your essence remains the same.

Think of today as a movie. Sometimes the pictures on the screen will be tragedy, sometimes comedy. But your essence is like the light from the projector. It remains the same even when there are no pictures flickering past.

OCTOBER

Of course there is no formula for success except, perhaps, an unconditional acceptance of life and what it brings.——ARTHUR RUBINSTEIN

SYMPTOMS AS UPPER LIMITS PHENOMENA

By now you may be familiar with the concept of the "upper limits problem," the tendency we humans have to bring ourselves back down after we've had a high time or a big win. For example, in one family Mom got a long-sought promotion. Shortly thereafter, one child developed a severe allergy to the local spring pollen, another started fighting after school, and Dad kept locking his keys in his car and calling his wife during her staff meetings. As they worked through this issue, they came to realize that each of them (including Mom) had specific fears about Mom's promotion. Would she surpass Dad in success? Would she spend less time with the kids? Would they end up having to move to a different house? Their symptoms—fighting, sneezing, losing keys—were a way to express those fears, and when the fears were acknowledged the symptoms disappeared.

■ A CONSCIOUS LIVING PRACTICE FOR TODAY ■

Tabulate your symptoms—physical illnesses, habits, relationship complaints. Take one or two of them and recall the last time you experienced them. Did they occur right after a period of having fun or feeling really good? If so, consider that they might be upper limits problems, ways of punishing yourself for feeling good. Consider other ways that might be easier on yourself.

OCTOBER 2

This is it!—FROM *LEAP OF FAITH* BY KENNY LOGGINS

YOUR WINDOWS OF DESTINY

Think of it:

A sprinting youngster skids to a halt, takes a jump shot at the buzzer, and ices the game.

A businessperson takes a deep breath and commits funds to a vision.

A field-goal kicker tunes out the roaring crowd, puts toe to pigskin, and clinches victory.

Two lovers let go of the past and make a commitment in the present.

A boardroom stalemate suddenly breaks through into resolution.

Everything important in life comes down to ten-second windows of opportunity where you move or stay put. If you move you might lose. If you don't you'll never know.

■ A CONSCIOUS LIVING PRACTICE FOR TODAY ■

As you go through your activities, be on the lookout for those tiny moments of opportunity that could change the course of your day and your life in a positive direction. Live in the question: What will it take for me to execute successfully in my windows of destiny?

OCTOBER 3

Growth is the only evidence of life.——CARDINAL NEWMAN

THE LEARNING PARADIGM

A learning paradigm offers certain advantages over a therapeutic or healing paradigm. In the latter paradigms, you need to identify something wrong with you before you can get better. While this viewpoint can be useful when you're sick, it's not very useful when you're not. A learning paradigm does not presume anything is wrong with you—it says simply that there are things you can learn to make your life more easeful and productive. The therapy paradigm often focuses on past events, presumably so a more positive present can be attained. While this may sometimes occur, the therapy paradigm often keeps people trapped in the past, perceiving themselves as victims. The learning paradigm invites you to take full responsibility for your life, make commitments in the present, practice those commitments, and identify goals for the future. The act of doing these things may pull past events to the surface, but they emerge in the context of a forward-looking journey to the future, not in a reference back to the past.

■ A CONSCIOUS LIVING PRACTICE FOR TODAY ■

Pause for a moment and ask yourself, "What do I most need to learn today?" Be open to any thoughts that come to mind. Today, pause frequently throughout your activities to wonder, "What do I most need to learn right now?"

OCTOBER 4

God knows I'm not the thing I should be,
Nor am I even the thing I could be.—ROBERT BURNS

STAYING COACHABLE

One of the most important things to remember in your journey of conscious living is: Stay coachable. Remember the tennis player Boris Becker? He won Wimbledon at the remarkable age of seventeen. The next year, though, he hardly got through the door. Guess what this extraordinarily talented youngster did after he became the youngest winner of the fabled tournament? He fired the coach who had helped him get there. Unbelievable as it may seem, that's just what he did. This awesomely gifted athlete displayed an equally awesome flaw. Perhaps he thought that since he'd won the biggest tournament at the youngest age of anyone in history, he didn't need much more coaching. Life then proceeded to kick this attitude off the court. Life often has a way of speaking to you gently if you're coachable but with brutal toughness if you're not.

■ A CONSCIOUS LIVING PRACTICE FOR TODAY ■

Pause to ask yourself, "Are there ways I could be more open to coaching?" Think of the people in your life. Are there ways you could make yourself more available to receive the wisdom they have to offer?

OCTOBER 5

The last thing one knows is what to put first.—BLAISE PASCAL

PUTTING YOUR CREATIVITY FIRST

Kathlyn, my wife and creative partner of two decades, made a creative breakthrough that she credits with revitalizing her life. Here's what happened, in her words: "One day I realized that when I didn't do the creative work I loved—writing poetry, doing movement improvisation, journaling—I was more critical of people around me. In other words, when I didn't access my creativity, I not only gave myself a hard time; I gave others a hard time, too. I decided to start putting my creative work first every day. Instead of paying bills or doing dishes first, and doing creative work later if I wasn't too tired, I reorganized my priorities. Creative work came first, and I did my chores later. The most amazing thing happened. First, of course, I got more creative work done, but I also had more energy later for chores. Everybody else in the family liked this new arrangement better, too. They got a new-and-improved model of Kathlyn, one who made good on her commitment to her creativity."

■ A CONSCIOUS LIVING PRACTICE FOR TODAY ■

As an experiment, change your priority of activities for a few days. Put your creative work first. If you want to write in your journal or do some painting or move to music, do a few minutes of it first thing in the day. Try this for a few days, taking note of any changes in your mood and energy level.

....

OCTOBER 6

All men by nature desire to know.—ARISTOTLE

WHAT YOU NEED TO LEARN

You never get to know what you need to learn until you open yourself to learning it. In other words, the moment you open yourself to learning, you find out what you need to learn. That's the way it has to work, because if you knew what you need to learn, you'd have already learned it. Most of you are not malicious—just defensive. Life tries to teach you something, and you say, "Yes, but I don't want to learn that right now." Or you say, "Yes, but I like my lessons delivered more gently." It's as if you think there are two faucets—one marked "Pleasure" and one marked "Pain." You think you can turn the Pleasure faucet on while leaving the other one off. There's only one faucet, though, and it's marked Consciousness. You turn it on and get to experience more life, which sometimes includes pain. Leave the faucet off, though, and you don't get to experience much at all except humdrum, tedium, and a slow leaking away of vital energy.

■ A CONSCIOUS LIVING PRACTICE FOR TODAY ■

Make a statement to yourself, to the universe around you, and even to others if you so choose. Say, "Today, I surrender myself completely to learning what I need to learn. I formally release my defensiveness, replacing it with a commitment to learning from every moment."

....

OCTOBER 7

An intense feeling carries with it its own universe, magnificent or
wretched as the case may be.—ALBERT CAMUS

EXPRESSING YOUR PASSION

What's your passion? I attended a Friday night potluck for the first time a while back. This particular potluck has been going on for many years, and unbeknownst to me, the traditional opening is for every person around the table to answer the question "What is your passion?" It was absolutely riveting to listen as one person after another responded to this question. For one person it was child-rearing; for another it was running a billion-dollar business.

What is your passion? Here are some clues that will help you to answer:

- Time passes quickly when you're engaged in this activity.
- The world—and your worries—disappear when you're doing it.
- Afterward, you feel exhilarated, full of emotional energy even if the activity has drained you physically.
- You can't imagine not having this activity in your life.
- Some of your fondest memories focus on engaging in this activity.
- A bad day engaged in this activity is better than a good day of most other things.

OCTOBER 8

I think I want to be mad for just one more minute, or maybe a week.
—TIMOTHY JOYCE, AGE FOUR

BREATHING IT OUT

Laura writes: He's sitting up on my bed, a solemn look on his face as he stares straight ahead. I ask what he's doing and he says, "I'm just being mad." After talking about why he's mad—and discovering that his anger is about something that happened days ago—I tell him that he can pretend his madness is right in his breath, and that if he opens his mouth and breathes out, he can get rid of that anger. I demonstrate, and smile to show him that I feel happy once the anger gets out. He watches me carefully and dubiously agrees that he's ready to lose the anger. He starts to imitate, and then stops.

"No," he says, folding his arms over his chest, a decision clearly formed now. "I think I want to be mad for just one more minute, or maybe a week."

Sometimes, even when you are given the chance to forgive, the tools and the opportunity to let go of the anger that builds up inside and tears you apart over time, bit by bit or in huge, biting chunks, you are not yet ready to free yourself from your anger. Better, then, to focus your attention on why you're holding on to your anger so carefully and jealously; better to pay attention to what's in it for you.

■ A CONSCIOUS LIVING PRACTICE FOR TODAY ■

Think about something you've been angry or resentful about recently—something you've not yet let go completely. Spend a few minutes wondering about your anger: its excuse (the outer name you give to the conflict), its real roots, and why you're not choosing to let it go yet.

- I say that my anger is about _____.
- My anger is really about _____.
- What I get from my anger is _____.

....

OCTOBER 9

Tell me whom you love, and I'll tell you who you are.——CREOLE PROVERB

SOUL-MATES

Laura writes: For a reason I haven't been able to identify, my seven-year-old has been somewhat obsessed with the concept of soul-mates lately. At dinner, driving in the car, in the quiet, before-sleep moments, he asks me about the whole idea: whether he's met his soul-mate yet (I tell him it's unlikely but possible, feeling vaguely wistful—remembering that in his first years, I, of course, was his soul-mate), how he'll know when he does. And then, as I fear, the question comes: *Mom? Who is your soul-mate?*

It is a dilemma in relationship. I have always tried to be clear and honest with my sons. Yet now I suspect that I know the answer he wants to hear me say.

"Who do you *think* is my soul-mate?" I ask, stalling for time.

"I was hoping," he says, "that you'd say you have one, but I don't think you do. You should, though."

"Yes," I answer slowly, smiling. "I should." And I should, and I *will,* I think to myself—the more conscious I have become, the more sure I am that a soul-mate is somewhere ahead of me. I continue, "I am surrounded by love, Christopher, and that is all I ask for right now." This seems to be enough for him—as it truly is enough for me right now—and he lets the question go for the time being. I am amazed once again at the depth of knowledge and knowing that exists between us. And I am saddened, too, because I can't give him what I know he knows doesn't exist—but what I think he must wish for. A soul-mate in every home, bliss in every heart. Someday, I promise him—and myself.

■ A CONSCIOUS LIVING PRACTICE FOR TODAY ■

Think about something that you've been sad about recently—something you've not yet let go completely. Spend a few minutes wondering about your sadness, and its real roots, and why you're not choosing to let it go yet.

....

OCTOBER 10

When three people call you an ass, put on a bridle.—SPANISH PROVERB

CRAZY-MAKING

George Bach, a psychologist who specializes in the study of conflict management, has identified seventeen—count 'em!—roles that people take in conflict, all of them passive-aggressive. This is not to suggest that some people don't handle conflict in a direct, assertive, and positive manner; instead, it is a commentary on the great lengths to which you will sometimes go to avoid open conflict. A number of these roles are built around the failure to take responsibility for your hostility, the refusal to acknowledge anger or resentment.

Are you an *avoider*, a *subject-changer*, a *joker*? In these roles, you deflect responsibility by dodging the subject when conflict arises. Are you a *trivial tyrannizer*, someone who expresses hostilities toward a partner by doing those little things—clipping toenails in the bed, belching loudly at a party—that drive your partner over the edge, while refusing to express your anger directly? Or, might you be a *pseudo-accommodator*, someone who appears to give in while carrying around a vast collection of slights and resentments, storing them up over time?

Begin to think about your style of conflict, how conflict makes you feel, and whether you're ready for something new, something direct, something satisfying and growth-oriented.

■ A CONSCIOUS LIVING PRACTICE FOR TODAY ■

With complete honesty, examine the role(s) you most often take in conflict and let yourself feel the fear and discomfort that conflict brings to you. Love your fear and your anxiety over conflict; being direct is not easy, but hiding behind the curtain of pretense is far more difficult.

....

OCTOBER 11

When we're afraid, everything rustles.—SOPHOCLES

NEW WAYS OF LOOKING AT FEAR

One of my favorite quotations is "Fear is excitement without the breath," attributed to the Gestalt therapist Fritz Perls. He is saying that the same body mechanisms that make you excited can make you scared when you forget to stay open and lively and full of breath. In other words, when you lose your commitment to full participation, you are likely to feel afraid. Then you will start looking for things to pin your fear on. And, of course, you will always find something. When you're afraid, you tend to look for the slightest little thing that will justify your giving up, pulling back.

Fear is naturally going to get stirred up when you move away from the known. As you open up your intuitive and creative powers—when you realize you have to make up life as you go—you're bound to feel afraid from time to time. It's nothing to be afraid of.

■ A CONSCIOUS LIVING PRACTICE FOR TODAY ■

As you go through this day, take note of your fear and what triggers it. Notice whether you get scared in response to physical events (such as cars backfiring) more or less than you do with social events (such as talking to someone you don't like). There are no right or wrong answers here . . . just begin to notice how your fear comes and goes.

....

OCTOBER 12

I thank God for my handicaps, for, through them, I have found myself, my work, and my God.—HELEN KELLER

THE GIFT OF BLINDNESS

Some years ago, while sitting in a restaurant, I noticed a man eating alone at the table next to mine. He looked radiantly happy, which was sufficiently unusual in itself, but I also realized he was blind. I could see his guide dog curled up napping at his feet. On the spur of the moment, I asked the man if I could join him. Soon we were deep in conversation. I remember two things from our time together. He told me that his blindness was the greatest gift he'd ever received in his life. When he'd rear-ended another car and was blinded instantly, it changed him overnight from a selfish drunk to a seeker of the truth. He said it awakened compassion and consciousness in him, two things he had never known about before. I was moved by this, but the second thing he told me left me in tears. He said he wasn't sure exactly what love was, because he'd never felt it as a child or been in love as a grown-up. But his feeling for his dog, he said, was the purest love he could imagine. They were linked together in a continuous circle of service and gratitude.

■ A CONSCIOUS LIVING PRACTICE FOR TODAY ■

Looking back over the powerfully painful moments of your life—your version of rear-ending a car and going blind—reflect on the gift that these experiences brought you. What did they allow you to feel that you might otherwise have remained unaware of?

OCTOBER 13

We carry with us the wonders we seek without us.—SIR THOMAS BROWNE

CULTIVATING CURIOSITY

Not long ago, I had the opportunity to talk to a well-known headhunter, a woman who'd made her fortune helping companies make inspired hiring decisions of top-level personnel. I asked her what her secret was. If she had two or three extremely qualified people, as she often did, how did she pick the one to recommend? She leaned over and whispered, "Curiosity. I look for the one with the most curiosity about everything."

"Curiosity?" I mused. "Tell me more."

She chuckled. "See, you're catching on already. The ones I hire are always more interested in learning than in proving how much they know."

■ A CONSCIOUS LIVING PRACTICE FOR TODAY ■

Today, make a commitment to curiosity. As you come into contact with various situations today, express curiosity. Avoid claiming to know. Go out of your way to set aside knowing for today, and instead use curiosity every step of the way.

....

OCTOBER 14

Each man must look to himself to teach him the meaning of life. It is not something discovered; it is something moulded.—ANTOINE DE SAINT-EXUPÉRY

CONFRONTING CHAOS

How do you deal with chaos? There is the inevitable tendency of things to fall apart, no matter how hard you try to keep up a discipline of conscious living. You'll be meditating and journaling and taking care of your body, and then things will go ahead and fall apart anyway. The ancient Hindu system describes three great universal forces: creating, maintaining, destroying. In other words, things will always be born, stay the same for a while, and fall into chaos. That's not a bad way of looking at things, because it takes off the pressure to create and maintain all the time. If you give yourself permission to fall apart now and then, you lighten up on yourself so that there's more room in you to accept the inevitable changing of circumstances.

■ A CONSCIOUS LIVING PRACTICE FOR TODAY ■

Ask yourself if you've been resisting chaos instead of acknowledging it as a valid part of life. Are there ways in which you've been clinging to certain ways of being instead of letting them fall away? If so, you may wish to open up to chaos and confusion for a while, giving yourself permission to let things change and disappear. The positive side of this is that for each falling away, something new is being born. For every chaos, a deeper level of creation and organization is trying to happen.

....

OCTOBER 15

My business is to create.——WILLIAM BLAKE

THINKING LIKE A GENIUS

How much time did you spend yesterday doing those activities at which you're a genius? How much time do you plan to spend today on those things?

Most of you, when asked these questions, reluctantly have to admit that you don't spend much if any time on your genius. In fact, most of you probably don't have a clear idea of what you're absolutely first-rate at. In my seminars, I spend a lot of time helping people identify their genius-level competencies. The first barrier I encounter is that many of them hesitate to admit that they're geniuses. Perhaps they think genius is weird or outside their reach or even dangerous. For starters, then, let's come up with a friendlier definition of genius. One friendly definition of genius is to think of it as those things you do that don't feel like work. When you're doing your genius—whether it's painting a picture or making a soup—you don't feel that you're working at it.

■ A CONSCIOUS LIVING PRACTICE FOR TODAY ■

Begin your embrace of genius by wondering what you're a genius at. Ask yourself two key questions: What do I love to do so much that I enter a timeless state while I'm doing it? And what am I better at than almost everyone I know? Be honest and forthright with yourself—you can be modest later.

The important thing is not to stop questioning.—ALBERT EINSTEIN

SEEK OUT A COACH OR MENTOR

One of the best ways to learn quickly on your path of conscious living is to model yourself after someone you admire. If you look around in your present life you'll probably find admirable people you have access to right now. I've found that people tend to be more generous with their time and advice than you might think if they are approached sincerely.

Early in my career I benefited enormously from coaches and mentors. In 1968, long before I'd ever published anything, I met a well-known poet and novelist in New Hampshire. Although there was a huge gap between our respective levels of the game, I transcended my fear and asked him if he would coach and mentor me in breaking into print. He was incredibly generous with his time and advice. In fact, he gave me several simple pieces of advice that have really allowed my career to flourish.

■ A CONSCIOUS LIVING PRACTICE FOR TODAY ■

Look around you today for potential coaches and mentors. Ask yourself, "Who is really leading the kind of life and doing the kind of work I admire?" If you spot some of these people, dial up the courage to ask them for coaching.

There are only two ways to live your life. One is as though nothing is a miracle. The other is as though everything is a miracle.—ALBERT EINSTEIN

OPENING TO ORDINARY MIRACLES

I have had the privilege of working with several dozen people after they have had major wake-up calls such as near-death accidents and life-threatening illnesses from which they've recovered. One thing I've noticed is that big, shocking events like those have a powerful effect on one's perception of the small moments of life. A wake-up call often seems to open us to the miraculousness of the ordinary. People become sensitive to sights, sounds, and smells that they formerly took for granted.

The question is: Can you greet the small moments of life as miracles, even before getting an unpleasant reminder to do so? With no prompting, can you learn to open yourself to the miracle of the air you breathe? The touch of skin? The sound of the wind? These are things people often start to notice after coming close to losing life.

■ A CONSCIOUS LIVING PRACTICE FOR TODAY ■

Pause half a minute to look around you right now. How many miracles can you appreciate without moving from this spot?

As you move through your day, take Einstein's advice and look at everything that comes your way as a miracle.

If you are lucky and work very hard, you may someday get to experience freedom from the known.—J. KRISHNAMURTI

LETTING GO OF KNOWING IT ALL

One of the chief problems that I've observed with living in an information-saturated age is that information itself becomes a potential addiction. I've noticed, during several silent retreats I've taken, that I go through a period of withdrawal from news, stock quotes, and sports scores. After about three days the urge to know it all begins to fade, but those first few days can be uncomfortable.

In conscious living workshops, I often have students get comfortable with saying the phrase "I don't know" over and over dozens of times. Each time they say it, I invite them to feel themselves getting more and more comfortable with not knowing. It's often illuminating for people to relax into conscious "not knowing." In a world in which being right is often an important value, it can be a real relief to feel okay about not knowing it all.

■ A CONSCIOUS LIVING PRACTICE FOR TODAY ■

Say the phrase "I don't know" ten to fifteen times. Each time you say it, accent a different word. Each time, pause for a few seconds to feel the quality of not knowing in your body.

As you move through this day, be sensitive to moments when you could use "I don't know" sincerely. Use it as often as you can, and notice the results.

If you are distressed by anything external, the pain is not due to the thing itself, but to your estimate of it; and this you have the power to revoke at any moment.
—MARCUS AURELIUS

THINKING MAKES IT SO

Aurelius wrote those words in a notebook he called "To Himself," and that I call "The Meditations of Marcus Aurelius." It's good to remember that this gentle man, forced by birth and a sense of duty to be both emperor and military chief of Rome, wrote them by night in his tent after fighting Huns all day. The external things that troubled him, then, were likely to be a lot harsher than many of the things that trouble you. I, for example, found my peace of mind riled today by a broken water heater, resulting in the lack of a hot shower. That's a much milder irritant than a barbarian invasion, yet your mind plays the same trick on you in either situation. There is the thing itself—invasion by Huns or broken water heater—and then there's your interpretation of it. One of the thinking flaws of the human mind is to confuse the unarguable reality of the event with feelings about it and estimations of it. Shakespeare later echoed this thought in his famous line "Nothing is good or bad but that our thinking makes it so."

■ A CONSCIOUS LIVING PRACTICE FOR TODAY ■

Begin to make distinctions between the reality of a given event—a toothache or a traffic light or a glitch at work—and your interpretation of it. Notice that the interpretation, no matter how accurate, is still only an interpretation.

OCTOBER 20

We do not see things as they are. We see them as we are.——THE TALMUD

SEEING THROUGH PROJECTION

One of the biggest breakthroughs you can make on the path of conscious living is to understand how projection works. Think of a movie projector shining through a film negative, projecting a picture on the big screen fifty feet away. Imagine what happens if a fly crawls across the surface of the projector's light. The audience laughs as it sees a magnified version of the fly on the movie screen. The same phenomenon plays havoc in daily life. Some small mood-shift will occur inside you, for whatever reason, and this tiny fly in your consciousness causes you to see the events of life differently. For example, you might be enjoying a wonderful meal at a four-star restaurant, when suddenly the person across the table tells you something you don't like. Now the food doesn't taste good, although nothing has changed but your own internal state.

It takes a genuine act of heroism to say, "The food's the same; I just don't taste so good right now."

■ A CONSCIOUS LIVING PRACTICE FOR TODAY ■

Every hour or so today, pause for a few seconds to ask yourself a question, "How is my mood affecting how I see the world right now?" Begin to develop a facility for noticing how your state of consciousness affects the movie that's playing on the big screen of your life.

OCTOBER 21

Failure is success if we learn from it.——MALCOLM FORBES

LEARNING FROM BARRIERS

Conscious living depends on the ability to live with a single question at hand: What can I learn from this? This question is particularly important when confronting barriers. By coincidence, just today I received two major rejections (a screenplay was rejected by two studios) and three major wins (foreign publishers made generous offers for rights to publish my books). If you greet each barrier with the wrong question—"What's wrong with me?" or "What's wrong with them?" —then you have to make each step of the process about what's wrong. This slows down the journey to a crawl, because then you have to greet each win with another set of useless questions—"What's right with me?" and "What's right with them?" What makes the journey smooth and fast is to greet each barrier (or each win) with a bow and an inquiry into what you can learn from it.

■ A CONSCIOUS LIVING PRACTICE FOR TODAY ■

Write the question "What can I learn from this?" on several pieces of paper or "sticky notes." Put these notes in prominent places where you'll see them as you go through the day. When you see them, take a moment to ask the question about the most recent event, positive or negative, that comes to mind.

No man is free who is not master of himself.—EPICTETUS

THE ONLY COMMITMENT THAT COUNTS

Epictetus was one of the greatest of all teachers of conscious living. He was born a slave but showed such brilliance that he not only was liberated but went on to found a school of philosophy in Rome. Trouble lay ahead, though, because a wave of religious fundamentalism swept through Rome, and all the philosophers had to leave town. He set up his school again in the hinterlands, and, fortunately, his students wrote down a lot of things he said.

Epictetus has a great many things to teach you, but one lesson stands out: If you are committed to the path of conscious living, you will do whatever it takes to make your journey. For Epictetus, the journey took him from being someone else's property to being entrusted with educating the children of the wealthy and powerful. Then it took him back to the countryside, on the wrong side of a wave of political conservatism. Throughout it all, his commitment seems never to have wavered, nor did the consistency of his message.

■ A CONSCIOUS LIVING PRACTICE FOR TODAY ■

Cut to what is essential. If you had to identify the three essential ingredients of a conscious relationship—those ingredients that you will not live without—what would they be? Once you've identified them, think about how far you're willing to travel to get them.

OCTOBER 23

Do not make yourself so big. You are not so small.—JEWISH PROVERB

PLEASING THE PLEASER

If you took all the approval-seekers out of the world, the population would drop by at least a fourth. A large number of you wear shrink-to-fit personalities, and are always on the lookout for what you could do to please others. The problem is, after you've made a few dozen chameleonlike changes in yourself during the course of the day, you may find when you go looking for your true self that there's nobody home.

There's a fine art to pleasing others without compromising yourself. There's nothing wrong with acting in ways that give pleasure to others, as long as you don't harm your own sense of being in the giving of pleasure. The moment you start seeking approval at the expense of yourself, though, you've made the first step in a slow process of eroding your own self-esteem.

■ A CONSCIOUS LIVING PRACTICE FOR TODAY ■

As you interact with people today, notice whether you compromise any of your values by trying to please them. Also, notice if you suspect others are compromising any of their values to please you.

....

OCTOBER 24

Life is short. Be swift to love!—HENRI AMIEL

ABANDONING HOPE

If you give up hope, you will likely find your life is infinitely richer. Here's why: When you live in hope, it's usually because you're avoiding reality. If you hope your partner will stop drinking, aren't you really afraid he or she won't? Aren't you really afraid to take decisive action to change the situation? If you keep hoping the drinking will stop, you get to avoid the truly hard work of actually handling the situation effectively. Hope becomes a drug or soporific to get you through the pain a little longer. Like all drugs, it comes with side effects. One of the main side effects is that you become a little numb, a little less alive. Hoping a situation will change keeps you at a distance from your true feelings—sadness, anger, fear. Each of these feelings is best appreciated up close. Feel them deeply, and they will cease to bother you. Hope they'll go away, and they'll bother you all day.

■ A CONSCIOUS LIVING PRACTICE FOR TODAY ■

Take ten seconds right now to notice what hope feels like to you. Savor the quality of hope. Notice how you might use it to avoid feeling deeper emotions that would be better approached directly. Notice if you use hope to block sadness, fear, or anger in particular.

....

OCTOBER 25

God respects me when I work, but he loves me when I sing.——RABINDRANATH TAGORE

BUSY-NESS AND STRUGGLE

Many people use being overly busy to avoid looking at key issues in their lives that need to be addressed directly. The same is often true for struggle. Many of you turn life into an unnecessary struggle, trying to prove to yourself and others how hard you're trying, when in reality all you're doing is burning up energy to avoid facing reality. The person on the path of conscious living treats busy-ness and struggle as addictions. If you give up the addiction, you'll finally get to address the issue that started you on the addiction. If you let go of struggle and quit over-committing yourself, you may find that you've been burning excess energy to keep your attention off truly important issues. Avoiding big issues such as expressing your creativity and handling painful relationship conflicts often provides the fuel for much unnecessary struggle and busy-ness.

■ A CONSCIOUS LIVING PRACTICE FOR TODAY ■

Pause for a moment to tune in to your body/mind. Check in and notice any sense of struggle in yourself. Notice the energy of busy-ness. Consciously let go of those for a moment and ask yourself a broad question: Do I use struggle and busy-ness to avoid handling aspects of my life that I ought to slow down and take a look at?

....

OCTOBER 26

Reason is also choice.—JOHN MILTON

RISK-TAKING

Babe Ruth said, "Don't let the fear of striking out hold you back." And he should know—in the course of hitting all those home runs he also struck out more than any other player. So what? When you think of Babe Ruth today, *strikeout* is not the first phrase that comes to mind. Babe Ruth and *home run* are forever entwined in our minds.

What would be your equivalent of hitting a home run? Would it be writing a poem or cooking a soup or getting into graduate school?

On the other hand, what would be your equivalent of striking out? Writing a poem nobody liked? Cooking a soup you weren't happy with? Getting rejected?

Notice that in each case, the strikeout can't even happen unless you swing. It's seldom the things you try and fail at that deeply trouble you late in your life—it's the things you never tried to do at all.

Make a list of your top-five "home runs." What would you accomplish if you swung big and connected?

....

OCTOBER 27

Then I saw you through myself, and found that we were identical.—FAKHR AD-DIN

RELATIONSHIP AS MIRROR

Many times in couples counseling I've seen people mired in conflict, only to discover after a session of therapy that they were actually sharing the same fear. For example, one person may be upset about money, while the other is upset about sex. Yet when they get beneath these surface struggles, they both find they are scared about some third issue they hadn't been aware of. Perhaps they were both afraid of life being out of control or afraid they would die without fulfilling their dreams. Because they did not know how to face this deep fear, they focused on a familiar squabble—sex or money. Once you get beneath the surface in any relationship, you may find you are much more like the other person than different.

■ A CONSCIOUS LIVING PRACTICE FOR TODAY ■

Think of someone with whom you struggle. Ask yourself: If I were not focusing on our differences, how am I exactly the same as him or her? Are we upset about the same thing, and only choosing to express it differently?

The environment is everything that isn't me.—ALBERT EINSTEIN

EVERY ACT OF HELPFULNESS IS A GIFT TO YOURSELF

A true fable: Once upon a time a depressed man called his friend, a therapist. He talked about his sadness, his anger, and his low station in life. The therapist listened. The man went on to describe how nobody liked him, he was underpaid, and his apartment was crummy. The therapist listened some more. Finally the man asked the therapist's advice. The therapist asked him if he had noticed anything in his neighborhood that needed fixing. After a long pause, the man said he'd noticed that the area around an elderly neighbor's front door needed sweeping. The therapist suggested the man go downstairs and sweep it carefully, and offered to wait on the phone until the man accomplished the task.

After ten minutes or so, the man came back and reported the task completed. There was a new energy and lilt in his voice. His depression had lifted through a simple act of service.

■ A CONSCIOUS LIVING PRACTICE FOR TODAY ■

Look for acts of service you could carry out today. Perhaps you'll see small ones, such as a pencil someone dropped on the floor that you could pick up and put away. Or perhaps you'll notice larger ones, such as a person in distress. Notice how you feel after you carry out each act.

....

OCTOBER 29

If you are unhappy, you are too high up in your mind.—CARL G. JUNG

THE BODY SENSATIONS OF HAPPINESS

One way of understanding Jung's quotation is to realize that concepts, which live "high up in the mind," are by nature cool and dry rather than hot and juicy. That's their strength and their weakness. You can plan a meal quickly because your conceptual mind works at lightning speed, but if you stay high in your mind when you eat that meal, you won't enjoy it and you might get indigestion. Your ability to savor life's experiences, whether food or love or music, comes from dropping down out of the sky of your mind onto the ground of your body.

That, of course, is where the pain is, too. When you come down out of the cool cerebral world into the heat of emotionality and sensuality, you descend through the same feelings that made you flee up into your mind in the first place. Once you learn how to breathe with your pain, though, there is a vibrant field of happiness to be savored.

■ A CONSCIOUS LIVING PRACTICE FOR TODAY ■

In your body, you can feel happiness. In your mind, you can think thoughts about your happiness. If you had to pick one, which would it be? Fortunately, you have the power to do both, so no choice is necessary. As you move through your day, notice that you can choose to focus on the body sensations of happiness. You may realize that they're there all the time—it just takes practice to feel them all the time.

....

OCTOBER 30

All thought is a feat of association: having what's in front of you bring up something in your mind that you almost didn't know you knew.
—ROBERT FROST

THE ONE PLACE YOU CAN'T SEE

If you took a driver's education course, you probably remember a lecture on the blind spot, the place behind you and off to the side where your rearview mirror doesn't work. You have to look in your mirror and glance backward over your shoulder if you are to get a panoramic view

of the situation. The same is true in living. Everybody has a blind spot
. . . or two or three. Your blind spot is the place where you can't see the
obvious. Some of the most gifted and talented people I've ever worked
with also had some of the biggest blind spots. When you think about
it, that's probably predictable. After all, the bigger the light, the bigger
the shadow it throws.

None of you needs to feel bad about your blind spots. When you get
defensive about them, they stay in place longer. What gets rid of your
blind spots—what gives you 360-degree vision—is openness to learning. The only thing you have to do is get willing to learn whatever you
need to learn.

■ A CONSCIOUS LIVING PRACTICE FOR TODAY ■

Pause ten seconds now to make a commitment for today. Say to
yourself, "I commit to learning from everyone and everything today."
Return to this commitment often throughout the day.

....

OCTOBER 31

Oh, EVOLVE.—BUMPER STICKER SEEN ON AN OLD VW BUG

THE ONLY ROAD

Laura writes: I'm driving to the mall, one of those big, sprawling
complexes that can sometimes induce a semi-panic attack if approached
in the wrong mind-set. I'm chattering away to a friend about a page of
Gay's I've recently read in which he talks about closet cleaning, ridding
oneself of that which one doesn't absolutely love. It's been a goal of mine
of late; I've promised myself that I will never again wear shoes that hurt
or fabric that doesn't feel fantastic against my skin. As a woman, I have
spent much of my life dressing to please others and being damn uncomfortable as a result. No more.

"You're going to be a granola-girl," my friend says, grinning. We both laugh, but she's admiring my goal. She rubs her feet (fortunately, I'm the driver) absentmindedly as we talk, saying that her feet always hurt from her shoes. I suggest she join me in this goal, and she shakes her head.

"I wouldn't know how to start being comfortable," she sighs.

I could think of a dozen suggestions, but what I hear in her voice is resistance, and so I don't make any comment. I feel saddened by her words, and strengthened in my own resolve.

■ A CONSCIOUS LIVING PRACTICE FOR TODAY ■

Earlier in your journey, you may have gone through your clothing and rid yourself of pieces you didn't like. Today, focus in on one thing that brings you physical discomfort: it may be a piece of clothing (shoes, a tie, a tight watch) or it may be something you do (standing slumped over, breathing shallowly, or tightening your neck with tension). Make a conscious commitment for the next twenty-four hours to evolve, to stop wearing this item or living this behavior. Make it your priority to be aware of the ways in which you side with your physical enemies, and betray the enemies; break camp and join yourself, letting go of discomfort and feeling the experience of being comfortable in your own body

NOVEMBER

NOVEMBER 1

I have never seen a greater monster or miracle in the world than myself.—MONTAIGNE

HAPPILY EVER AFTER

There is a cartoon panel in a book I've taught from that shows a mother sitting at the bedside of her young child, reading a storybook. The cover of the book says *Modern Fairy Tales.* The mother is saying: "And the prince and princess learned to lower their expectations and lived reasonably contentedly ever after. The end."

Many of you watched the fairy-tale wedding of Great Britain's Prince Charles and the late Princess Diana; Laura, who at the time was the same age as Diana, writes: I watched it with chills because it looked like the fairy tales I'd heard all of my life—maybe they could actually be true! Girl meets prince, girl marries prince, and girl (magically transformed into a princess) and prince ride off in a glass coach into a life of hazy splendor. Who could help hearing, though, about the demise of the fairy tale: crying scenes at posh ski resorts, suicide attempts, binging and purging, cold distance, infidelity? So maybe, many of us thought, there are no fairy-tale endings after all.

What a shock when you learn that real life intrudes on even the most magical of fairy tales. He belches in front of her friends; she is a closet smoker; he leers at other women in front of her; she doesn't want to have sex so much once the children are born. And so on.

My hope for you on your conscious journey is one of reconciliation: I wish for you a healthy dose of the struggle that gives long-term love its depth, laced with the laughter and intimacy that layer partnership with so much richness.

■ A CONSCIOUS LIVING PRACTICE FOR TODAY ■

What is your fairy tale? What did you once think your marriage or long-term relationship would be like? And how has that rose-colored vision changed because of reality? Spend a few moments thinking of the fantasy versus the reality, and then answer for yourself the questions below.

- What don't I have that I always thought I'd have?
- What do I have that I never expected?
- How far apart are my fantasy and reality?

....

NOVEMBER 2

Every child is an artist. The problem is how to remain an artist once he grows up.
—PABLO PICASSO

BE CREATIVE

I passed a man sweeping the sidewalks in a business district recently. The man was wearing the uniform of a maintenance worker, but he had on a T-shirt that said "Be Creative" on the front and "No Matter What You're Doing" on the back. It gave pause for thought.

What if you invested every action you take with lovingness and creativity? What if sweeping sidewalks, repairing burst water heaters, reading to a child, cooking a meal, writing a report for work, and even sleeping were conscious actions filled from the well of your creativity?

This is how I try to live, and it has introduced a remarkable level of comfort and excitement and magic to my life. I encourage you to make the same commitment, to decide today that it is not enough to simply live; instead, you are going to live large, live exuberantly, live creatively, investing the smallest of your actions with the richness of your creativity.

How to start? I'll begin with just a few simple suggestions.

- Dress creatively and comfortably, in "eye easy," body-affirming clothing.

- Be conscious of your breathing throughout the day; make sure that you are breathing deeply, from your diaphragm, the core of your creative self.
- Be conscious: as you begin any action, ask yourself how you can invest it with your own style and creativity. Perhaps this means singing as you cook, or perhaps it means a reframing, reminding yourself that cooking does not have to be a chore, it can be a gift of your love and yourself.

■ A CONSCIOUS LIVING PRACTICE FOR TODAY ■

Identify one activity that is repetitive and boring in your life, such as preparing daily meals, cleaning up after your family, driving a carpool, or sitting through meetings at work. Open your mind and your creative self: as is so often said now in business, "think out of the box" for a moment. What one simple change can you make to invest this routine and repetitive activity with creativity? Be aware of how your experience changes once you layer creativity on this activity or behavior.

....

NOVEMBER 3

*In every winter's heart there is a quivering spring
and behind the veil of each night there is a smiling dawn.*—KAHLIL GIBRAN

LETTING IN THE THIEVES

One of our neighbors is in the process of building a second-story deck onto the back of his house. We got a view into not only the deck-building process but something far more buried in this neighbor's heart and experience when he began trying to decide, during a discussion with us, whether to put stairs on the deck. He was concerned that it would make his house too accessible for thieves.

As he listed the pros and cons, we began to believe that he was really talking about a deeper level of fear for his safety. A single man who jumps from one short-term, intense relationship to another, and has for the twenty or so years he's been an adult, he was trying to come up with a way in which he could gird and guard himself against the possible inroads someone might make into his heart.

We decided to take a risk, not knowing the man very well, and point out our observations. His eyes instantly glittered with tears, and we told him that we were glad to have raised the issue about his loneliness and self-protection.

"You made me cry," he said, sounding astounded. "I haven't cried since I was a boy."

"That's great!" we rejoiced. "You let someone in!" He shook his head at his wacky neighbors and went off to make his decision alone.

At this moment, looking out of the window in our writing room, we can see the deck as it nears completion; the stairs rise up to join the deck flooring, and our neighbor has built sunburst patterns into the railings all the way up the stairs.

■ A CONSCIOUS LIVING PRACTICE FOR TODAY ■

Think about something you do to keep others at a distance. Perhaps you're super-competent so that no one can see your need; perhaps you're just the opposite, asking others to take care of you as a way of keeping your relationships unbalanced, unequal. Zero in on one behavior that is symptomatic of your distancing needs, and let go of it today. Ask for help, drop something—literally or figuratively—tell someone the heart of how you feel, cry, let go of being "on" in your persona and instead just be. Just be.

The giving of love is an education in itself.—ELEANOR ROOSEVELT

CREATING A WORLD-VIEW

You have two great tasks in your life: to live in peace within yourself and to live in harmony with the people around you. If you do not find peace within yourself, nothing you accomplish will feel satisfying. You can blanket yourself with the finest of material belongings, surround yourself with perfect children and trophy partners, be at the top of your profession . . . and it will be of no import whatsoever. Similarly, if you do not connect and live in harmony with others, you miss the very essence of life: affiliation, connectedness, the giving and receiving of love.

Once you are in harmony internally and externally, you can join together into an ecological action—a balance with the world around you, relational and physical—that springs upward from a center of wholeness. Only then, I believe, will we preserve the harmony of the earth and keep it well for our children.

What exists inside of you is inextricably linked, like a deep root system, to the well-being of the planet. You cannot save the integrity of the planet on which you live if you cannot even save yourself.

■ A CONSCIOUS LIVING PRACTICE FOR TODAY ■

Spend fifteen or twenty minutes outside today, weather permitting, or, if not, plant yourself comfortably in front of a window. Look around and take in the majestic, incredible harmony of the earth: animals living in a system of balance, trees and grass and flowers and plants rising up out of the richness of the earth, the sweet air filled with life-supporting oxygen, the sky stretching out for miles. Feel your tininess first: feel how small you are in the greater system of life. It is humbling and affirming to see yourself as a small part of such an unimaginably large system of life. And now feel your largeness: feel the space you occupy, the breaths you take, the way that your body feels as it is anchored to this one spot of earth. Feel the connectedness between you and your world, our world. Know that every breath, every action, has some lasting effect on our world. Tread gently.

......

NOVEMBER 5

To appreciate heaven well, 'tis good for a man to have fifteen minutes of hell.
—WILL CARLTON

COLD SHOWERS

I returned from a speaking engagement at midnight, after a grueling four-hour flight, yearning for a hot shower and a good snooze. My wife was out of town, so I let myself in, dropped my luggage, and trudged to the bathroom to take my long-awaited shower. There, I was greeted with cold water: In my absence the water heater had broken.

The next day I called my niece, Laura, and in the course of the conversation I lapsed into griping about my water-heater problems. Tongue in cheek, she suggested I lovingly embrace my cold shower and let it be a source of spiritual teaching for me. "Don't use all that conscious living stuff on me," I said, picking up on her gentle cue to lighten up. "This is serious. This is my water heater!"

Sometimes water heaters break, cars sputter to a halt on the way to job interviews, people career around us giving us the finger when we're prudently obeying the speed limit. That's life on planet Earth sometimes, and what can we do about it?

Have a few good friends, for one thing. Have a few people we can call who'll gently remind us, as Laura did, that people did just fine without hot showers for thousands of years, and to be grateful, as I was, when the plumber came (on a Sunday, no less) and restored order to my universe.

Today, take note of things that go wrong. Jot them down. Pause during the day and look over your list, reframing each one. Find another way to look at each troubling situation. Be your own best friend.

....

NOVEMBER 6

I am made of the same stuff as everything else in the world.
I am the same as the oak leaf and the earthworm and the sky beyond.
It is all one thing, and I am a part of it.

THE HOLY REAL

On my journey, I have discovered a radical surprise: any and every aspect of reality is sacred. If you go deeply into what is real, you will find all the transcendence you crave deep in your soul. Those things that are traditionally considered holy—angels, ghosts, visions of heaven—are all magnificent to those who perceive them. Yet each is arguable, so arguable that wars have been fought over the reality of them. You are going to enter the cathedral of the real, however.

If you can focus on reality instead of fantasy, you can feel spirituality moving in your body rather than simply thinking about it.

■ A CONSCIOUS LIVING PRACTICE FOR TODAY ■

Breathe. Just breathe. Feel your breath as it enters and exits your body, allowing it to come from deep in your belly, and allowing it to fill your lungs with clean, affirming oxygen. Slowly dismantle your protective walls, the ones that keep you in fantasy instead of reality. You will not win the lottery today, Mr. or Ms. Right is not knocking on the door, and your boss is not going to call you into the office to tell you that you've received a promotion—you are not—not today, anyway—going to be promoted to the position of king or queen of the world. Just breathe. What about reality—this moment, right here, right now—is enough? What about this moment *isn't* enough? You're alive, are you not?

....

NOVEMBER 7

I put myself on an opinion diet, in which I avoided forming new opinions and quit defending the ones I had. My wife liked this diet a lot—she thought the new slimmer version of my previously fat head was much more becoming.

KNOWING AND KNOWING

As a human being, I suffer from a grand illusion: I think that safety comes from contracting around my opinions, making them right and then defending them. The problem with doing life this way is that you then must clump together with other people who share the same opinions, seeking the larger safety of the herd. You'd think you'd have happiness and harmony, then, with everyone seeing the world the same way, but it actually works in an opposite way. Soon, everyone unites under an authority and troops off to do battle with another group holding different opinions. Even if there is no other group, battles break out within the group: little cartels and secret societies and factions and cliques form. You must, after all, have some way to whittle away your time between wars.

With your head buried in the sand of reality (which is, in truth, only *your* imperfect interpretation of reality), you're in an ideal position when the universe comes along, as it invariably does, to kick you in the keister.

Most of the difficulties you experience in life are your own way of teaching yourself this principle: *Take all of life as it comes. Feel it. Breathe with it. Let it go.*

Think about a kick you've recently received from the universe. Maybe you were driving along in traffic, singing to the radio, and nearly had an accident. What was the universe trying to tell you? Perhaps you heard some information from a friend that your partner shared with the friend but not you. Again, what message and learning might you take from this occurrence? Open up how you see and interpret reality.

- The kick was _____.
- The message was _____.

....

NOVEMBER 8

Men at some times are masters of their fates:
The fault, dear Brutus, is not in our stars,
But in ourselves, that we are underlings.——WILLIAM SHAKESPEARE

WHO ARE YOU?

You must be wary not to embrace any belief that takes you out of oneness with the universe. The moment you do so, you render your force-field dense and impermeable. The moment you begin believing you are a fallen angel or a risen ape or a reincarnated llama, you cease resonating with the wholeness of all. Then adversity begins and will not cease until you again embrace oneness.

Oneness with the universe means seeing the ways in which we are all connected—and we *are all connected*. The jeans you are wearing, stitched by a young woman in Guatemala, the computer on which I type, created into being by many minds and hands, the person who laid down the asphalt upon which you drive each day—each action connects you to another action and, most important, to another person. We're in this together, as the saying goes, and recognizing that connection will help you to see your place in the universe.

I find that when I acknowledge my connection to others—sending a note to the friendly woman at the flower store who always has a kind remark, stopping off for a cup of cappuccino and dropping it by a friend's workplace for him, including people half the world away, ones you don't know but with whom you share the universe, in your thoughts or prayers . . . all are ways of acknowledging your ultimate affiliation, and the ways in which we are forever linked, forever dependent on one another.

■ A CONSCIOUS LIVING PRACTICE FOR TODAY ■

Today, identify someone who you wouldn't typically thank . . . someone who would never expect a thank-you from you, but who impacts positively on your life. Sit down with a postcard or notepaper and tell the person how she or he makes a difference to you . . . and then send the note. If this sounds Pollyannish, consider this: you walk out to the mailbox today, and in with all those never-ending bills is a note from your mail carrier. *Just wanted to let you know*, it says, *that you made my week yesterday when you smiled and sympathized with how hard my job must be in this weather. It meant the world to me.*

....

NOVEMBER 9

Joy is not in things. It is in us.—RICHARD WAGNER

A CARDINAL LESSON

One of the key lessons of conscious living goes something like this: Get your priorities straight. Focus first on who you are inside, then let your actions come out of this wellspring of self-knowledge. Don't focus on external appearances or achievements while your inner life languishes.

In counseling sessions, I have worked with many high achievers who have won big awards, only to find themselves feeling depressed a day or two later. When I was twenty-five, I set myself the goal of getting my Ph.D. when I was twenty-eight. I put in three years of intense work, during which I barely nodded at my emotions, my dreams, my relationships. I received my doctorate within ten days of my twenty-ninth birthday, but the day after, I could hardly get out of bed. As I lay there, wondering why I felt so numb, I realized it was because I'd thrown myself out of balance through my effort, and now that it was over I wasn't sure I could get back in harmony again.

Thanks to the resilience of human beings, it's never as hard as it looks, but for a while I wondered if I would ever feel a flow of ease inside me again. Looking back, I'm glad I did the necessary work, but I wonder if I could have done it in a way that kept me more in touch with my inner world.

■ A CONSCIOUS LIVING PRACTICE FOR TODAY ■

As you go through your day today, pause to ask yourself now and then: Could this be easier? Could I do this in a way that lets me stay in touch with who I am inside?

....

NOVEMBER 10

I have one request: may I never use my reason against truth.—ELIE WIESEL

GAMES PEOPLE PLAY

Laura writes: Running on a lake path recently, I encountered a past lover. The relationship had ended very oddly; the lover had moved (which I'd been expecting) but had not contacted me with his new phone number or address. It was one of those nightmare-quality experiences. I could have located him, obviously, but his total disconnection from me, without warning, seemed like a clear message. I have wondered, sometimes with great sadness, why he never called to say goodbye or to officially end what was, in truth, never much more than an affectionate physical relationship. His action had felt hostile, understandably, and I had searched myself for a time to see if I had given him reason to fear ending directly what we had openly agreed would one day end when we met closer partners. I felt clear with myself that I had not caused his behavior, and at that point, I let it go.

With some hesitation, I fell into step beside him. "Why'd you do that?" I asked. After all this time, my question felt more curious than anything else.

He didn't answer for a time, and we ran together, our hard breathing and the sound of our feet hitting the path the only noises around. Finally, he answered. "I was afraid to hurt you."

I laughed. "I was touched by your kindness," I said, rolling my eyes.

He laughed, too. I figured he was remembering my occasional lapse into sarcasm. "Yeah, well," he said. "Smart women, dumb choices." That was an old line—a joke between us back then—when I had struggled with the rightness of being in a relationship that wasn't "going anywhere."

Both of us laughed at that line, and then he shrugged, and we exchanged awkward good-byes, and I picked up the pace and moved ahead down the path. He'd never been as good a runner as I was; I remembered, as I rounded the lake and glanced over my shoulder, glimpsing him far behind, that he'd never been able to keep up.

■ A CONSCIOUS LIVING PRACTICE FOR TODAY ■

People do things that hurt you. The issue, of course, is what you contribute. Think on a recent instance in which you've been hurt in an interaction. What part did you play?

Generally music feedeth that disposition of the spirits which it findeth.
—FRANCIS BACON

INTO THE MYSTIC

There are times—hours, days, weeks—when I live in perfect harmony with the universe. This, I believe, is the presence of love in my life.

When you allow yourself to stop resisting reality, instead moving in a state of grace with the workings of the world around you, allowing yourself to feel your deep connection to every aspect of the world, large and small, you become most open to love's power and to love's potential.

The energy you spend trying to resist and redefine the universe, which time and again proves itself most unwilling to adapt itself to your whims, is instead channeled inward to become the fullest, truest realization of yourself. Songwriter and poet Joe Cocker sings about "the mystic," which I think of as the state of grace that occurs when love is not only the actualization of truth and connection between two people but also the actualization of truth and connection between each of us—in our heartbreaking smallness and our infinite grandness—and the universe we occupy.

■ A CONSCIOUS LIVING PRACTICE FOR TODAY ■

You may be a person who carefully turns off lights as you leave a room, only runs water when your hands are actually in the water, and so on. Or perhaps you are less conscious of saving resources and energy. Take a hint from the first type of person and apply it for today to your personal life. Think of a way in which you can turn off the taps on your personal energy in an area where it is being wasted, recognizing that it is a limited resource. You may set a limit with someone, or you may set a limit with yourself, but identify one specific way in which you can reserve your resources for something more worthwhile to you. Focus on your feelings as you try this experiment.

....

NOVEMBER 12

In peace, sons bury their fathers; in war, fathers bury their sons.—HERODOTUS

ACTING OUTSIDE OF THE HEART

I have been aware, lately, of the horrifying stories of children shooting other children in schools. I have been talking to others, over the past few days, about resisting reality and working against the universe, and it is in situations like these, so inexplicable and so terrifying, that it is most difficult to accept life as it is. I want to offer you a twist on accepting reality, however; I want to assure you that accepting reality does not mean shrugging your shoulders and assuming that you have no control or power over events around you. To the contrary, you have tremendous power; by accepting reality, you are simply saying that you must work with rather than against the forces that exist.

The example in the schools is relevant. It would be possible, I suppose, to simply shake my head and comment on the state of adolescence these days . . . and then move on, forgetting about it. However, if you are guided by love and by a commitment to making a difference in the universe, an event this horrifying might instead spur you to do something—anything—that could change future events. You might decide to use your counseling expertise to provide community education about the warning signs of violence. You might use your strong sadness closer to home, talking freely and honestly with your children, educating them about paying attention to threats that other children make.

When someone acts outside of the heart as you know it, committing an act so violent and so damaging to your sense of the world, conscious living means taking in that act, accepting that it occurred, and accepting that each of us owns at least some small part of it. This is not about guilt. This is about responsibility. The difference is larger than the universe, and the results of taking this level of responsibility are universe-changing.

■ A CONSCIOUS LIVING PRACTICE FOR TODAY ■

Today, read the headline news in the paper or online or listen to news radio for the big stories. Choose one story that hits you on an emotional level, something that might normally make you feel helpless, and make a commitment to yourself to accept your responsibility for this event (it happened in your world, my world) and to act on that. Your action may be small, it may be large; the essential is action.

....

NOVEMBER 13

Wisdom is knowing what to do next. Virtue is doing it.—DAVID STARR JORDAN

CULTIVATING GENEROSITY

Many people think of generosity as something they would do after becoming prosperous. Actually, it works the other way around. If you lead with generosity—rather than waiting for it to come to you—you'll be rewarded with much more than financial prosperity. Think of generosity first in the basic processes of daily life. Imagine, for example, what it feels like to be listened to generously. When you speak, a generous listener pays careful attention not only to the words you say but to the feelings beneath those words. You are able to speak without interruption, because the generous listener, before replying, extends his or her listening into the silence beyond your words. Now turn the tables. Imagine yourself as a generous listener, a philanthropist of loving attention. Just as John D. Rockefeller would give a shiny new dime to children who came up to him, give a shiny new space of open listening to people who come into your presence. Generous listening is a huge first step toward generating a generous spirit.

■ A CONSCIOUS LIVING PRACTICE FOR TODAY ■

Today, focus on a single dimension of listening: interruption. See if you can go an entire day without interrupting anyone. Discover the people you have the most trouble listening to without interruption.

....

NOVEMBER 14

A man there was they called him mad. The more he gave the more he had.
—JOHN BUNYAN

CONSCIOUS PHILANTHROPY

Almost everyone who embarks on the journey of conscious living eventually becomes a philanthropist. One person may philanthropize to the tune of millions, another to the tune of dozens of dollars, but the principle they follow is the same: The more you give, the more you get back. This is not to say that philanthropists give with the sole intention of getting back—it only means that a basic principle of life is that you get back from the universe what you put into it. If you open your heart and your pockets abundantly to the world, you are likely to be showered with abundance in return.

As you mature on the path of conscious living, there is a tendency toward simpler living. At the same time, as wisdom grows, you tend to reap more financial rewards. Often you end up with a wonderful problem: how to give away more and more. Then, since you tend to get back what you give, this problem gets bigger and bigger and bigger. Pretty soon, you may be wrestling every moment with the problem of how to receive and give vast amounts of love and money. Human beings love to wrestle with problems, so if you're going to be doing it anyway, this is not such a bad problem.

■ **A CONSCIOUS LIVING PRACTICE FOR TODAY** ■

Select an amount to give away this year. Do your best to arrive at the amount by some means other than calculating a percentage of your income. In other words, make your giving proactive and not tied to your income.

....

NOVEMBER 15

If you treat men the way they are, you never improve them.
If you treat them the way you want them to be, you do.—GOETHE

OVERCOMING OLD HURTS

In conscious living, old hurts can and should be brought to mind and body in order to face them and accept them and complete whatever unfinished business there may be. The reason is that old hurts, if hidden from the light of consciousness, often cause barriers to love and success in the present. If you get your tonsils taken out, a time will come, perhaps a day or two later, when swallowing hurts terribly. In that moment, a wise doctor or nurse will counsel you to reach for chewing gum instead of a painkiller. The reason is that the muscles around the wound must be stretched and used in order to restore the flow of circulation to them.

The same idea applies to old emotional hurts. You need to air them out, letting them move and breathe, so they don't freeze into long-term contraction.

Think about any areas of your life that are not working as well as you'd like. As you focus on an area, ask yourself two questions: Are there wounds I haven't recovered from that are affecting this area of my life? If so, how might I heal those wounds?

NOVEMBER 16

As you walk, eat, and travel, be where you are.—BUDDHA

THIS PRECIOUS MOMENT

Read what several teachers of conscious living have said about time and forward movement, and about paying attention to the present:

I am just going to leap into the dark.—FRANÇOIS RABELAIS

There is a time for some things, and a time for all things;
a time for great things, and a time for small things.
—MIGUEL DE CERVANTES

Life can only take place in the present moment. If we lose the present moment, we lose life.—BUDDHA

■ A CONSCIOUS LIVING PRACTICE FOR TODAY ■

Pause for ten seconds and savor this precious moment: This is it! As you pass through this day, savor often the present reality, no matter how important or seemingly unimportant.

NOVEMBER 17

The thoughts that come often unsought, and, as it were,
drop into the mind, are commonly the most valuable of any we have.—JOHN LOCKE

UPGRADING THOUGHT

More than a hundred years ago the great American psychologist William James said that the most important discovery of his generation was that "a human being can alter his life by altering his quality of mind." Written several thousand years before our time, the Upanishads contains the same idea: "What you think about, that you become." Earl Nightingale, a few decades ago, read more than a hundred classics of psychological and spiritual growth, and found one idea they had in common: The quality of your life can be changed by upgrading the quality of your thoughts.

It's a powerful notion, and one you can readily check out for yourself. In fact, it's only through experimentation that you can prove that this timeless concept really works.

■ A CONSCIOUS LIVING PRACTICE FOR TODAY ■

Right this moment, pick an area of your life that you have some negative thoughts about. Perhaps it is a relationship or your car or your job. Consciously drop one positive new thought about this area into your thoughtstream. Just one new positive thought. Then watch closely over the next few days to discover if there's a change in the outer circumstances.

Great services are not canceled by one act or by one single error.——BENJAMIN DISRAELI

BENEFITING FROM ADVERSITY

For thousands of years, teachers of conscious living have been telling us that we grow through adversity. A Chinese proverb says, "The gem cannot be polished without friction," while a German proverb echoes a similar thought: "Who has never tasted the bitter can never know the sweet." Yet it's always hard to remember these wise words at the moment you're actually going through adversity. When fear comes up strongly in your body, it often shuts down the philosophical center of your brain for a while. It's hard to philosophize about rhinoceroses when there's one actually chasing you. Your first task is always to acknowledge your present "feeling state," whether it's fear or anger or joy. Then you can recommit to learning through adversity.

You can also surround yourself with friends who know how to ask the right questions. In times of adversity, your best friends ask, "What can you learn from this?" Your false friends ask, "Why is the world treating you this way?"

■ A CONSCIOUS LIVING PRACTICE FOR TODAY ■

Pause to wonder about your present life. Think of where you are currently experiencing adversity. Focus on one area and ask, "What am I needing to learn that I've created this adversity for?"

Don't ever take a fence down until
you know why it was put up.——ROBERT FROST

TRANSCENDING ADVERSITY

Some lessons must be learned through direct experience. You cannot learn to make a great soup by reading a cookbook, nor can you become a great lover from watching a video. Other lessons can and should be learned by pure wisdom rather than raw experience. Looking back over the great leaps forward of your life, you may notice that you've grown enormously through adversity. However, you also may notice that sometimes a little bit of wisdom could have prevented some unpleasant raw experience. The country singer Loretta Lynn once said, "I'd never heard of birth control until I was pregnant with my fourth child."

There is an intention you can set that will open the maximum "growth space" for you. The intention is to learn those things from experience that absolutely must be learned that way, and to learn those things by wisdom that can be learned that way. While you can't learn to cook soup by wisdom, neither do you need to spill it on yourself repeatedly if you can learn, by wisdom, to use a spoon instead of a fork.

■ A CONSCIOUS LIVING PRACTICE FOR TODAY ■

Say the following commitment in your mind: *I commit to learning from experience when necessary, and to learning from wisdom when possible. I commit to learning from wisdom when doing so can prevent unnecessary pain to me and others.*

NOVEMBER 20

. . . from cradle to tomb, it's not that long a stay.——FROM THE MUSICAL *CABARET*

KEEPING TIME

There is a time paradox that you all live with. From the perspective of infinity, you have all the time in the world. Even though the dinosaurs were on earth over a hundred million years, it seems as though they were here and gone in the wink of an eye. From the perspective of right now, you also have all the time in the world. As long as you're fully in the present, you seem to exist in a timeless zone. But from the perspective of an insurance agent, you have a little more than 25,000 days. The agent can run a finger down the actuarial chart and tell you with amazing accuracy how long you'll be around. Did you have healthy grandparents? If yes, add a couple of thousand days. Do you smoke? If yes, subtract a bunch.

Part of being human is embracing the paradox of time——focusing on the infinite inside you and around you, yet being solidly grounded in the reality of life as a finite flicker in eternity. In conscious living, you learn to feel the radiant glow of the eternal while at the same time showing up on time for appointments. Neither one is more important than the other.

■ A CONSCIOUS LIVING PRACTICE FOR TODAY ■

Take a deep breath and commit yourself to living fully this moment, this day. Remember that this moment is the only one you have, and that you need to recommit to being fully present in it nearly as often as you breathe.

NOVEMBER 21

Where no hope is left, is left no fear.—JOHN MILTON

THROUGH THE GATE OF FEAR, INTO THE ZONE OF FREEDOM

It's not unusual for you to feel fear when you take responsibility for your life. Hundreds of times in therapy I've watched people catch a wave of fear just as they've stepped into full responsibility for something. Often, for example, people will get scared just before making a commitment to something big, like getting married or jumping into a new job.

Why does this happen?

It's because the moment you take responsibility for something, you tap into the creative forces of the universe. The universe has no problem creating an oak tree or a volcano or a dinosaur. It creates things effortlessly, because it is the source of creation. When you think of yourself as a victim, you lose sight that you are part of universal creation. You are the universe, too. People often get scared of all that power, and cower in an it's-bigger-than-me relationship with the universe. When you're feeling that you don't belong in the universe or that it's you against the universe, time to take a few deep breaths into your fear and remember that there's only one thing in the universe—whatever you want to call that one thing—and we're all made of it.

■ A CONSCIOUS LIVING PRACTICE FOR TODAY ■

Take a few deep breaths into your fear zone: for most of you that's in the belly. Then ask yourself, "What can I take responsibility for today?"

He who would do good to another, must do it in minute particulars.—ANONYMOUS

WHEN YOU DROP SOMETHING, PICK IT UP

I made a simple but life-changing discovery some years back: I was walking across my living room when I noticed a paper clip on the floor. I could feel part of me wanting to ignore it and part of me wanting to stop and pick it up. Pausing for a few seconds, I tuned in to both feelings. Suddenly I realized that for most of my life I had operated from an "I'll take care of it later" mentality, which pushed things out of my awareness that actually could be handled on the spot. So I reached down and picked up the paper clip. Instantly I felt lighter and more relaxed, as if part of my mind could be free to focus on more important things. This small incident led to dozens more observations over the next few months. Many times I caught myself noticing something and simultaneously trying to pretend I hadn't noticed it. As I gradually trained myself to handle things on the spot rather than taking care of them later, I felt a great deal more energy and ability to focus on the present.

■ A CONSCIOUS LIVING PRACTICE FOR TODAY ■

Put your attention on incompletions today. As you go through your day, notice any incidents of leaving things until later that could be done on the spot. Experiment with doing them as soon as you notice them, and notice the effects of these actions on your mind and body.

The pause—that impressive silence, that eloquent silence, that geometrically progressive silence which often achieves a desired effect where no combination of words, howsoever felicitous, could accomplish it.—MARK TWAIN

DAILY QUIET TIME

Almost everyone who journeys along the path of conscious living discovers the value of solitude. If you have found the joys of daily quiet time for yourself, congratulations. If you have yet to savor this treasure, put it high atop your priority list.

You can do a formal meditation practice in which you dedicate an hour or so a day to quieting your mind and body. Or you can do something simple and informal, such as a few minutes of breathing fresh air in the morning. On two occasions in the past week, for example, I have stopped by the ocean in the midst of a busy errand run to enjoy the sound of the waves and the sea breezes. Ten minutes of seaside solitude was all it took for me to recharge the flagging batteries and renew contact with nature.

■ A CONSCIOUS LIVING PRACTICE FOR TODAY ■

Today, pause at least once in your rounds to take some quiet time. Pull your car under a tree and sit for a few minutes, or get up a few minutes earlier for a morning communion with nature. Notice how your minutes of solitude affect the hours of your day.

NOVEMBER 24

'Tis not love's going hurts my days,
But that it went in little ways.—EDNA ST. VINCENT MILLAY

MAKING CONTACT

I was on a business trip to Manhattan a few years ago when, as I was paying my bill at a restaurant, the cashier remarked that I must be from out of town. I admitted that I was and asked her how she'd spotted me. "Easy," she said. "You smiled and made eye contact with me as you were paying your bill."

■ A CONSCIOUS LIVING PRACTICE FOR TODAY ■

As you go through this day, take time to make genuine connections with people you meet. Make eye contact with people who pass through your life. Reach out to them with your generous attention.

NOVEMBER 25

Life consists in what a man is thinking of all day.—RALPH WALDO EMERSON

THE VALUE OF DOING NOTHING

The resistance of boredom is a powerful driving force in many people's lives. To avoid boredom, many of us haunt the malls, eat things when we're not hungry, chatter about things we know nothing of to people we don't care about. Once, on a trip to India, I learned an important lesson about boredom. I stayed for several days at a tiny ashram in the foothills of the Himalayas. There was absolutely nothing to do there. The guru didn't even believe in yoga or meditation, considering them a futile use of time. Instead, he encouraged us to do nothing, to let ourselves be bored, and especially to let go of any notion of improvement. It was a brilliant spiritual ploy. After a couple of days of frantic urges to do something—anything!—my mind completely let go, allowing me to experience a depth of peace I had only glimpsed before.

■ A CONSCIOUS LIVING PRACTICE FOR TODAY ■

Sit for ten minutes today, doing nothing. If you find yourself doing nothing for some reason, such as to notice what your mind does when you do nothing, stop doing that and simply do nothing.

....

NOVEMBER 26

I find even bad people good, if I am good enough.—LAO-TZU

LISTENING TO FIX

Most of you listen through a "fix it" filter when you listen to others. If a friend starts to tell you about some problem, you listen to it with intent to fix. If a pain develops in your shoulder, you tune in to it with intent to fix. What would happen if you let go of your "fix it" mentality for a little while? Would you fall apart? Probably not. Very likely you would fall together.

If you listened generously to others, you would not approach others as problems to be fixed but as open spaces of creative possibility. Perhaps then you would create a world in which much less needed to be fixed.

■ A CONSCIOUS LIVING PRACTICE FOR TODAY ■

As you interact with people today, do your best to do unfiltered listening. Listen to people purely, as if you had no agenda other than to appreciate what they say.

Little do men perceive what solitude is, and how far it extendeth. For a crowd is not company, and faces are but a gallery of pictures, and talk but a tinkling cymbal, where there is no love.—FRANCIS BACON

HONORING YOUR INFLUENCES

Appreciation is one of the main operating tools of conscious living. Whatever you encounter is something you, for some reason, need to encounter. Therefore, you might as well appreciate it. While it's tempting to do the opposite of appreciating—resisting the heck out of it—there is really no point. Eventually you will have to look into why you've brought a given situation into your life, so you may as well do it sooner than later.

The same is true for the positive influences that have brought you to where you are in life. If you look back over your life, you'll realize that there are people without whose influence you would never be where you are today. Honor yourself for bringing them into your life, too.

■ A CONSCIOUS LIVING PRACTICE FOR TODAY ■

Pause for a moment to appreciate people in your past who helped you get where you are. Begin with silent appeciations—"telepathic" telegrams. Then, if you can, express verbal or written appreciation to people. Develop the habit of appreciating people on a regular basis, and notice what happens in your life as a result.

Once upon a time a man whose ax was missing suspected his neighbor's son. The boy walked like a thief, looked like a thief, and spoke like a thief. But the man found his ax while digging in the valley, and next time he saw his neighbor's son, he walked, looked, and spoke like any other child.—LAO-TZU

A LESSON BY THE FIREPLACE

Of all the lessons of conscious living, clearing up projection may bring you the most rapid relief from upset. I had a personal experience of the power of projection a while back. I was in front of the fireplace talking to Kathlyn. Without realizing it, I was leaning to one side, propped up at an uncomfortable angle by my arm. As the conversation continued, my side of the conversation grew more and more negative. Soon I was focusing entirely on the pain of human existence and my paltry role in it. After a while my mate gently pointed out the tone of my words and inquired, "Could it be that it's your arm hurting and not the world?" I changed my position and suddenly the world looked like a much better place.

■ A CONSCIOUS LIVING PRACTICE FOR TODAY ■

When you find yourself shifting toward a negative mood, change your position—either the position you're occupying in your mind or the actual physical position of your body. Notice if your mood changes.

NOVEMBER 29

Fear is excitement without the breath.—FRITZ PERLS

BREATHING SPACES

Conscious breathing is one of the most powerful techniques of conscious living. It also has the great benefit of being absolutely free. Pausing to take a few deep breaths at key times during the day can make your whole life run more smoothly. It only takes a few healthy breaths to pep you up when you're tired or calm you down when you're feeling overly buzzed.

Breathing is hooked up to the voluntary and the involuntary nervous system: you can take a deep breath on purpose, or you can forget about your breathing all night long while you sleep. For this reason, breathing makes a perfect place to focus your attention during your year of living consciously.

■ A CONSCIOUS LIVING PRACTICE FOR TODAY ■

Today, use your breath to create space in places where you might otherwise crowd yourself or others. After others speak, for example, pause to take a breath before replying. When you're feeling an emotion, pause to breathe a few times with the intention of letting yourself feel it completely. Give yourself and others room to breathe.

Every real thought on every real subject knocks the wind out of somebody or other.
—THE HOLY REAL

CONSCIOUS DRIVING

I tend to be a cautious driver (but also one who's never had an accident, knock on wood!). I was on a beautiful winding country road where the speed limits were marked at 20 around curves and 35 on the straight parts. A double yellow line indicated that it wasn't safe to pass. I was cruising along, enjoying the scenery, when a driver came up behind me and stayed about five feet from my back bumper. Looking in the mirror, I could see he was angry. His jaw muscles were bunched up and he made some "hurry-up" gestures at me. Finally he roared around me, in violation of the yellow lines, and disappeared off into the distance. About fifteen miles down the road I came around a curve and saw his car literally sitting on its roof in a ditch. Several people had gathered to help, and a policeman was waving people around. As I crept past I saw the driver standing near the car. This time he had a very different expression on his face. He looked shaken but also transcendent, as if grateful to be alive. I've always wondered if he could have learned the lesson in a gentler way.

■ A CONSCIOUS LIVING PRACTICE FOR TODAY ■

Ask yourself, "Are there any lessons in my life I could be learning in gentler ways? What would I need to do to learn my life lessons as gently as possible?"

DECEMBER

DECEMBER 1

Fear is the thief of dreams.—ANONYMOUS

SHARPENING YOUR INTUITION

One of the most frequently asked questions at lectures I give on conscious living is "How do I know the difference between intuition and the voice of my ego?" For example, you might have an inner prompting to buy a new sports car. How do you know this impulse is based on a genuine intuition? How do you know that you're not just feeding your sense of self-importance, the part of you that would be pumped up by being seen around town in a fancy car?

One way to discern intuition from ego is by tuning in to the presence of fear in your body. Often, when the ego's in charge, you'll notice that you're feeling a lack of something, such as self-esteem, and this lack will usually be accompanied by fear. Genuine intuition does not usually come with fear attached. I say usually, though, because intuition is far from being an exact science, and your own experimentation is as good as any expert's advice.

■ A CONSCIOUS LIVING PRACTICE FOR TODAY ■

Tune in to your inner-body sensations for a moment. Fear is usually a speedy, queasy feeling in your belly, often accompanied by tight stomach muscles. Do you feel even a subtle signal of it at this moment? Tune in throughout the day, beginning to notice what situations trigger it.

DECEMBER 2

When a true genius appears in the world you may know him by this sign, that the dunces are all in confederacy against him.——JONATHAN SWIFT

THE GIFT OF RIDICULE

Ridicule should be worn by creative people as a badge of honor, because so many of the inventions you take for granted were greeted with derision by the ignorant. You may never have heard of Clarence Saunders, a grocer who was ridiculed far and wide by his peers for an idea he tried out around 1920. Up until then you presented your list to a clerk, who went back to the shelves and brought your groceries to you. Saunders started allowing shoppers to wander among the shelves and pick out their own stuff. Lo and behold, he discovered that this freedom inspired shoppers to buy more than they had on their list. Almost before his critics had stopped laughing, Saunders had a chain of forty stores dedicated to "freedom shopping."

■ A CONSCIOUS LIVING PRACTICE FOR TODAY ■

As you move through your day, look for ways in which you could create more freedom in your life. Is there an invention or a change you could make that would create more ease?

....

DECEMBER 3

Shall I compare thee to a summer's day?——WILLIAM SHAKESPEARE

WINTER'S TALES

A few years ago my wife and I began a new tradition: reading aloud to each other. Both of us had been blessed with family members who read aloud to us as children, and we had continued the tradition by reading aloud to our own children. Why not read aloud to each other?

We began with Shakespeare's sonnets and then went on to other poets of then and now. It became a treasured part of our day, usually practiced before bedtime on winter evenings.

Then we discovered another reading treat. At one of our workshops, we happened to mention one of our favorite novels, Gabriel Garcia Marquez's magical book *One Hundred Years of Solitude.* Only a few people had read it, so we recommended it heartily to those who hadn't. Then, we asked the participants to tell us their favorite books. It turned out we hadn't read many of their favorites. We made a list and began reading our way through it. Now, it's become a tradition to ask people to tell us their favorite book so we can add it to our list.

■ A CONSCIOUS LIVING PRACTICE FOR TODAY ■

Make a list of your top-five favorite books. Then, offer to trade lists with a few of your friends. Read their favorites . . . there's no surer way to get to know someone better than to live with one of their treasured books for a few days or weeks.

....

DECEMBER 4

There are no facts, only interpretations.—FRIEDRICH NIETZSCHE

LIFE, LIBERTY, AND A REALLY SWEET BOSS

Are you entitled to be surrounded by people who treat you really well? By people who are unfailingly kind to you? Absolutely not. There is no guarantee, and this is particularly true in the workplace, that you will be treated well. You do not have control over how others behave; what you do have control over is how you respond, and this includes what you decide to tolerate.

Laura writes: I have been blessed with wonderful bosses (including, for a long time, my mother), but I once had a boss who had minimal experience, and even less natural skill, in employer-employee human relations. I remember this boss castigating me once (for something that I had, indeed, done wrong, so the content of the reprimand was accurate and deserved). The person stood in a central office and, with raised voice, shook a stack of papers at me and reprimanded me in front of several other employees. I apologized for what I had done, but the shame and humiliation stayed with me afterward. Others suggested I should quit (I didn't feel like I could, financially), or at least that I should confront the boss and tell her how off-base she'd been, castigating me in front of others. I chose not to address the issue; based on dealings with this person, I had decided I was unlikely to create any change even if I spoke with her, and I chose to direct my energies elsewhere. The one thing I remember carrying away from the experience, though, was a philosophical sense of shoulder-shrugging; you're not given the inalienable right to be surrounded by people who approach the world as you do. Once I accepted the basic unfairness that can sometimes crop up, it was simple to let it go and move forward in meeting my own goals rather than wasting energy railing against reality and trying to change what was unwilling to be changed in the universe.

■ A CONSCIOUS LIVING PRACTICE FOR TODAY ■

Think of a situation in which you feel that you were unfairly treated—perhaps at work. Consider the energy you put into feeling put upon and angry. Ask yourself the following questions—and the next time such a situation occurs, try *acceptance* instead of *resistance*. Let yourself feel what a difference it makes.

- When the situation occurred, my primary feelings were
  _____.
- Even though I didn't do it, I imagined _____.
- I could have used my unproductive energy to instead _____.

Life is action and passion; therefore, it is required of a man that he should share the passion and action of the time, at peril of being judged not to have lived.
—OLIVER WENDELL HOLMES

FLOODING AND FLOWING

When feelings flood, it is usually because you have built them up—picture a vast reservoir of feeling that has been dammed up inside of you, and, at some point, the damn dam breaks. Woe to anyone in the path of the powerful floodwaters of your unchecked feelings. You can choose to harness this energy—a topic I've been discussing in great detail for a number of days now—and direct it toward a *flow of feeling*, which washes everything clean, rather than a *flood* bent on destruction.

Interpersonal communication scholars recommend the following approach for dealing with feelings that may seem overwhelming or difficult:

Step One:	Describe the behavior you observed.
Step Two:	Interpret the behavior you observed.
Step Three:	Share how you feel as a result of the behavior.
Step Four:	Discuss the consequences of the behavior.
Step Five:	Discuss your intentions as a result of the behavior.

For the next five days, I will discuss each step in detail, walking you through the why and the how of each part of this approach to conflict management and "feeling sharing." For today, commit to learning and practicing this new way of honoring your feelings.

You have been learning a great deal, I hope, over the months that you've been on your journey with me. Today, commit to another learning, one that I have committed to totally, and one that can have life-changing implications because of how well it helps you to share "big" feelings and confront difficult relational issues.

Commitment: *I commit to learning how to honor my feelings and perceptions and those of the others with whom I have relationship.*

....

DECEMBER 6

Life, as it is called, is for most of us one long postponement.—HENRY MILLER

DESCRIBING BEHAVIOR

Yesterday I introduced the idea of flooding or flowing; today I begin with the five-step process of expressing feelings that result from another's behavior, feelings that may seem overwhelming when they are still swirling around within the finite space of your internal self. Once your feelings are allowed out into the largeness of the universe, you are likely to find that they are more manageable—not less important but smaller. The first step in the process of setting free your feelings is to describe the behavior that you believe precipitated those feelings. Note: the example situation I will use for the next five days is presented just below.

The situation: Your partner has a habit of looking other men or women up and down slowly and sexually, and oftentimes commenting to you on some physical feature that she or he finds attractive.

Step One: Describing the Behavior. You are in charge, here. How you approach this will likely determine the outcome. What you must be aware of is that your feelings are involved in this, and that they're likely to show themselves right away. However, it's your job to avoid that; Step Three addresses feelings, but in Step One all you are doing is objectively describing your partner's behavior.

I noticed you watching that woman as she walked by, and then you just commented on what nice legs she has.

Observe: Do not *judge* ("I noticed you *ogling* that woman") and do not *interpret* ("you must not find me attractive") and do not *threaten* ("if you do that again, so help me _____"). Simply describe what you observe.

■ A CONSCIOUS LIVING PRACTICE FOR TODAY ■

Practice describing behaviors you observe—without judgment of those behaviors. When your partner slams a door, you can observe (to yourself; this is practice), "I heard the door slam when you went outside." When your child pouts, you will observe, "I notice that your lips are sticking out and you are frowning." It can be difficult to leave off the judgments, but it's essential. It sometimes helps if you imagine yourself writing an introduction to a newspaper article: all you are addressing so far, though, is the *what,* and *when.* No *how* or *why* for today!

....

DECEMBER 7

The only real voyage of discovery consists not in seeking new landscapes but in having new eyes.—MARCEL PROUST

INTERPRETING BEHAVIOR

Once you have described a behavior you've observed, eliminating judgment from your description, the next step is to interpret that behavior. Keep in mind that this is your interpretation—which means that it may or may not be valid for the person with whom you are communicating. Interpreting, too, is nonjudgmental, in a sense. While there is always judgment involved in deciding what someone's intent is, you are taking full responsibility for your perception, and thus you are not accusing or blaming the other of having certain motives; you are simply sharing with your partner your impressions of the *why* I didn't address yesterday.

What You've Said So Far: I noticed you watching that woman as she walked by, and then you just commented on what nice legs she has.

Step Two: Interpreting the Behavior. We all make many assumptions about why others do the things they do, and often we give these assumptions little thought; we just take it for granted that we know the motivations of others. This is so often incorrect. Step Two allows you to share your assumptions, but it also creates a context in which you are making it clear that you are not at all certain that you corner the market on perception.

> When you watched her, and then when you commented on her legs, I assumed that you were feeling attracted to her.

Observe: Again, do not *judge* ("You shouldn't be doing that when you're married," for example). You also made it clear, by using the word *assumed*, that you take ownership of your perceptions, rather than defining the world and insisting that your definition is necessarily correct.

■ A CONSCIOUS LIVING PRACTICE FOR TODAY ■

Practice interpreting behaviors you observe—again, without judgment of those behaviors. When your partner slams a door, you can interpret (still to yourself), "I assumed you were angry." When your child pouts, you might interpret, "I'm thinking you might be disappointed about not going with me." Today is the *why!*

Oh for a life of sensations rather than of thoughts!—JOHN KEATS

LINKING FEELINGS TO EXPERIENCE

Now that you have described and interpreted a behavior you've observed, keeping in mind to eliminate judgment from both steps, the next thing you're going to do is to identify how you're feeling as the result of the behavior and your interpretation of the behavior. Remember, it is your interpretation of the behavior that is creating how you feel. We choose how we perceive certain events, and if this is true, it stands to reason that we also choose, then, how we respond emotionally. By keeping out judgment, and by describing your feelings, you are creating a non-defensive communication environment. You are acknowledging to your partner that she or he has an impact on you, but you are taking responsibility for how you perceive and respond to your partner.

What You've Said So Far: I noticed you watching that woman as she walked by and then you just commented on what nice legs she has. When you watched her, and then when you commented on her legs, I assumed that you were feeling attracted to her.

Step Three: Linking Your Feelings. Now that you have set up the situation, describing to your partner the *when* ("when you did such and such") and the *what* (the behavior) and the *why* (your interpretation), it is time to share with your partner *how* you're feeling about what took place. Before you begin this process, you will want to honor yourself and your feelings by taking the time to search your heart and listen to your own voice; if you listen respectfully, your heart will tell you how you feel.

I felt insecure and sad, because I've been feeling unattractive lately. I felt scared that I might be losing you to someone you find more attractive.

Observe: You're not pulling any punches. This is a painful, deep, essence-level disclosure about your deepest feelings—and as such, this is a relationship builder of the highest sort. This time, you're guarding against judging yourself. Your feelings are your facts: no apologies necessary ("I know I shouldn't feel this way," for instance, is judgmental and does not honor your essence).

■ A CONSCIOUS LIVING PRACTICE FOR TODAY ■

Practice identifying your core feelings. You'll find yourself going through layers (anger, resentment) to get to the essence (fear, insecurity, abandonment). Allow yourself to go all the way down into the depths of the *how:* how you feel.

....

DECEMBER 9

If way to the Better there be,
it exacts a full look at the Worst.—THOMAS HARDY

BEHAVIOR AND CONSEQUENCES

You have described and interpreted a behavior you've observed, and you have shared the feelings that you are having as a result of the behavior or interaction. Step Four is to discuss the consequences of the behavior. This does not mean to threaten, or even to reasonably share what will happen if the behavior occurs again. The consequences are internal; what you are going to be searching for inside of yourself, and then sharing with your partner, is the behaviors with which you are likely to respond as a result of the event that took place. This requires paying close attention to your history, your patterns, and your own sometimes dysfunctional or unproductive ways of relating to others.

What You've Said So Far: I noticed you watching that woman as she walked by and then you just commented on what nice legs she has.

When you watched her, and then when you commented on her legs, I assumed that you were feeling attracted to her. I felt insecure and sad, because I've been feeling unattractive lately. I felt scared that I might be losing you to someone you find more attractive.

Step Four: Stating Consequences. Now you've shared the *who*, the *what*, the *why*, and the *how*, it is time to share with your partner another *when* and *what*: you're going to more fully explain *what* you are inclined to do *when* your partner behaves in this way.

I find myself withdrawing from you to avoid these feelings, and I also notice that I avoid doing things in public with you so I don't have to face this.

Observe: Again, this is essence-level communication. You're taking responsibility for your behavior, and you're telling your partner what impact she or he has on you. It doesn't get much more honest than this.

■ A CONSCIOUS LIVING PRACTICE FOR TODAY ■

Recognize the things you do that are linked to the behavior of others. Take full responsibility, and peel back the layers of blame and rationalization to face head-on the ways in which you participate in conflict and in perpetuating behaviors others exhibit that create problems for you. Whose team are you on?

....

DECEMBER 10

Is not this the true romantic feeling—not to desire to escape life,
but to prevent life from escaping you?—THOMAS WOLFE

INTENTIONS

You're almost there! You've described, interpreted, and linked a behavior to your feelings. You've also shared with your partner the ways in which you are likely to respond to the behavior that took place. The final step in this process involves your intentions: what you intend to do about the behavior, and, more important, your own relationship with the behavior.

What You've Said So Far: I noticed you watching that woman as she walked by and then you just commented on what nice legs she has. When you watched her, and then when you commented on her legs, I assumed that you were feeling attracted to her. I felt insecure and sad, because I've been feeling unattractive lately. I felt scared that I might be losing you to someone you find more attractive. I find myself withdrawing from you to avoid these feelings, and I also notice that I avoid doing things in public with you so I don't have to face this.

Step Five: Stating Intentions. The final step can be seen as the "so what?" of the process. If after stating the "what you've said so far" section above someone said, "So what?" to you, your intentions are what you would provide as an answer.

So, I'd like to talk about what you're thinking when you do that, and about whether you're aware of how painful it is for me. You see, I'd really like to keep spending time with you out in public, just without the pain.

Observe: You've stated your intentions, or what you want (to discuss it, to know whether this is about attraction for your partner, to know whether your partner realizes how painful this is for you; you've also stated the intention of wanting to continue to be together in public). Look through this process carefully; there is no judgment, and this is why it works.

■ A CONSCIOUS LIVING PRACTICE FOR TODAY ■

Today, practice intentions: practice requesting things from your partner without judging and without blaming. Practice, too, leaving behind the guilt at your want, and while you're at it, practice silencing that voice inside of you that may be saying you want too much. This is your life, and this is your love. What is too much?

··

After the game, the king and pawn go into the same box.——ITALIAN PROVERB

LOOKING FOR DIFFERENCES

Our brains are highly skilled at looking for differences. Just to walk across the room, for example, your brain has to make a multitude of decisions about one thing being different from another. To take a step, your brain has to notice the difference between your foot and the floor and then do it all over again a second later. You could even say that we evolved because of millions of years of noticing differences.

One of the biggest problems in relationships is the tendency to focus on differences rather than similarities. In couples counseling, I've noticed that a couple may have a thousand similarities but spend their time and energy fighting about a few differences. It helps to realize that you come wired from the factory to notice differences. Once you realize that this tendency is part of your inherited physiology, you don't need to take it as seriously. You can put more of your energy into celebrating similarities.

■ A CONSCIOUS LIVING PRACTICE FOR TODAY ■

In your day's activities, go in search of similarities. As you encounter a coworker, for example, ask yourself, "How am I like this person?" Take time to celebrate the way you and others are just alike.

There are times I think I am not sure of something which I absolutely know.—
MONGKUT, KING OF SIAM

VISUALIZATION AND EMOTIONALIZATION

By now you've probably discovered the power of visualization in your life. You know how to create pictures in your mind of what you want to appear in your life. It's a useful skill to have, because most of us come from a background in which we went around creating negative pictures in our minds unconsciously. Far better to create conscious pictures of what you want rather than spending the same energy creating unconscious pictures of what you don't.

Now let's go one step further to use emotions to empower your visualizations. Next time you visualize something you want to create, turn on your positive emotions and feel it, too. In addition to picturing a new job, feel yourself doing it. If you want to manifest a new Ferrari, see it in your mind's eye and feel yourself behind the wheel of it, enjoying the roar of the engine and the wind in your hair.

■ A CONSCIOUS LIVING PRACTICE FOR TODAY ■

Think of something you want to create in your life. It can be a material object or a relationship quality or a spiritual dimension. See it in your mind, and at the same time feel it in your body. Use your feelings to give support to the pictures in your mind.

Our fears are more numerous than our dangers, and we suffer more in our imagination than in reality.—SENECA

REAL THREATS, IMAGINARY FEARS

Nature has gifted you (or cursed you, depending on how you look at it) with an exquisitely sensitive nervous system. Sometimes it may seem like a very nervous system, indeed. Laboratory studies show that your "fear machinery" can fire off at the tiniest of provocations—even the thought of a feared object, such as a snake, can cause your heart rate to pump up and your hands to get clammy. That's why, in learning to live consciously, it's a good idea to put a lot of your attention on noticing which of your fears are based on imaginary events and which are based on real events.

Real threats can be dealt with or endured. Imaginary threats cannot be dealt with or endured, because they're not real. The only move that can help with imaginary threats is to regard them as what they are—imaginary.

■ A CONSCIOUS LIVING PRACTICE FOR TODAY ■

Make a study today of the things that upset you, rile you up, and scare you. Notice how many of them take place between your ears and how many take place out in the world around you.

....

What if I should discover that the poorest of the beggars and the most impudent of offenders are all in me, and that I stand in need of the alms of my own kindness; that I myself am the enemy that must be loved—what then?—CARL G. JUNG

LOVING THE INFERNAL INTERNAL

A friend of mine is a prominent philanthropist who, years ago, was convicted of a white-collar crime and spent two years in a penitentiary.

According to him, it was the best thing that could have happened to him. It transformed him into a generous and warmhearted person, open to love and creativity. In prison, he learned to meditate, a practice he still does faithfully every day. Best of all, he says, it taught him to love his inner prisoner, that part of him (and, most likely, all of you) that thought of himself as a victim who was bent on getting even with the world. He points out that many people spend years in therapy without getting such a remarkable result.

■ A CONSCIOUS LIVING PRACTICE FOR TODAY ■

Take time out right now for ten seconds of pure love for your inner victim, the part of you that feels entitled to . . . everything! Give it a loving retirement celebration right now, and let it have the day off.

....

DECEMBER 15
Determine that the thing can and shall be done, and then we shall find the way.
—ABRAHAM LINCOLN

UNDER CONTROL

Laura writes: About ten years ago, I had a serious car accident. Sitting at a red light in a small car, I was hit by a tractor-toting truck. For months after the accident, I was anxious, and, although I still drove, I found it to be a fearsome activity. It wasn't until I accepted the accident—the meaning of the accident—that my comfort returned. In my case, acceptance sounded something like this: *Bad things can happen randomly. I might die in the next hour. I am going to die at some point, no doubt about it. Until then, I am going to live in recognition of these truths. Every day is going to be lived with the recognition that it may be my last; because of that, I don't have time for anything less than truth and love and real connection.*

Now, with time and distance on my side, I can muse on it with more of a philosophical view; the thing that is most striking to me is that I often insisted, back then, that I had things under control, and the accident illustrated that control had me. It's an interesting phrase, *under control.* You are, in fact, under it, and your job is to shake it off, emerge out into life where the unpredictable, the awful, the magnificent happens, humbling you and encouraging you to let go of your attempts at controlling the universe. All you have to do is pay attention and you'll hear the message: *Control is a tough mistress. Better to lose her and find your sense of abandon and joy instead.*

◼ A CONSCIOUS LIVING PRACTICE FOR TODAY ◼

Identify an area in your life where you try to exert rigid control—often with poor results. Today, trying letting go at three different levels. To let go, what you will do is repeat an affirmation, feeling yourself as you release your grip on something that cannot be gripped.

• Mind: I recognize with my logical self that the universe has its reasons.
• Heart: I recognize with my emotional self that the universe has its reasons.
• Body: I recognize with my physical self that the universe has its reasons.

DECEMBER 16

Courage is the price that life exacts for granting peace.—AMELIA EARHART

APPRECIATE RICHLY

From thousands of years of dealing with adversity, our minds have become finely honed to look for what's wrong. A parent can wake up at the tiniest whimper of the baby in the next room, and a driver can detect the subtle shimmy that may become a full-fledged rattle if unattended. All day and all night you are keenly attuned to what might be going wrong, especially when things are going well.

For this reason, it takes a heroic commitment on your part to focus on what's right. Focusing on what's right is a key skill of conscious living. What you focus on tends to grow, so if you want to have more joy in your relationships, you need to focus on the joy you have. If you want more creativity in your life, you need to focus on the creative gifts you enjoy.

It's as simple as that.

■ A CONSCIOUS LIVING PRACTICE FOR TODAY ■

Looking around you this moment, appreciate the things you see. As you go through your day, pause now and then to take stock of the richness of your life. Appreciate more, and notice that, as if by magic, you have more to appreciate.

....

DECEMBER 17

People hardly ever make use of the freedom they have; for example, freedom of thought; instead they demand freedom of speech as a compensation.—SØREN KIERKEGAARD

FEAR AND MOVING FORWARD

Laura wrote to tell me of a friend's discovery: The friend was ending a marriage, and said she wasn't afraid of losing the relationship or supporting her kids or even being alone at night. She said the one thing she feared was trying to remember how to connect with people again. She said she had "relationship laryngitis," which she defined as an inability to remember how to do small talk, carry on a conversation, make dates, and so forth. One night at a pub, she looked around the table and saw a woman of nearly fifty who was getting divorced after twenty-six years of marriage, a man who'd never lived with anyone except his parents, a couple who was newly dating, and a woman who was single and in her thirties and deeply wanted children.

Suddenly she realized: We all have the same issue to face. Every one of us is always confronted with the task of connecting with people in an authentic way. She felt her whole body relax as she knew she wasn't alone anymore.

■ A CONSCIOUS LIVING PRACTICE FOR TODAY ■

Today, muster the courage to connect with someone you haven't made contact with ever or for a long time. Reach out to a person—a new acquaintance or an estranged one—and see what happens.

....

DECEMBER 18

A man, Sir, should keep his friendship in constant repair.—SAMUEL JOHNSON

HAVING A HONEY

Laura writes: My family is fortunate to have had the same babysitter for almost four years. Two of my sons can't even remember another sitter. It's not just the long-standing nature of the relationship that's important, of course; "Honey," our sitter, is a part of the family. She's a child at heart and an adult at mind, the ideal combination to make children feel happy and parents feel safe. Christopher, my oldest son, introduces her: "This is Honey. She's not just our friend. She's family." And this is the magic of Honey—she is one of those people who is so enmeshed, in all the right ways, in our lives, that she is, indeed, family. She is *acquired* family, the kind that I hope you also have in your circle of friends.

You are born into whatever family creates you. This is not about choice. As children, you often absorb the ways of that family in ways that stay with you forever—although you do have choices about what you keep and what you discard as you get older. But friends, friends are all about choice, about the freedom to surround yourself with the kind of people you want in your life. There is nothing artificial, nothing forced or contrived, in the best of your friendships; they are freely chosen, freely continued, and they make you larger than you might otherwise be.

■ A CONSCIOUS LIVING PRACTICE FOR TODAY ■

Today, think about the circle of friends in your life: new friends and old, familiar friends. They are woven into the fabric of your experience, knowing things about you, about the way you see the world. Take a moment to appreciate your family of friends; they are a gift you give yourself every day.

....

DECEMBER 19

If stars appeared only one night every thousand years, how we would marvel and adore them.—RALPH WALDO EMERSON

RIDE WITH THE WIND

On a beautiful, sunny Memorial Day, my niece, Laura, took her three kids on a "venture," as her youngest boy called it, and sent me an e-mail about it: Riding in a water-taxi to Ft. McHenry, my middle child was heavily asleep against me, my youngest was making hilarious nonsensical comments, and my oldest was chattering with a new friend he'd just made on the boat. I relaxed, as best one can knowing that water, the parent's potential enemy, is only a few feet away. So much of parenting—even our parenting of ourselves—seems like running an obstacle course. The dangers! It's hard to remember to live in the moment and let my guard down. For a moment, though, as the sun shimmers on the blonde hair of these three lives so precious to me, I let go and appreciate how easy and simple life is. It's up to me to keep them safe, but it's also up to me to let them (and me!) ride with the wind in our hair.

Try on a guiding idea in your mind: *I ride through life in safety, and I also give myself absolute freedom to ride with joy, with the wind in my hair.*

....

DECEMBER 20

When one door of happiness closes, another opens; but often we look so long at the closed door that we do not see the one which has been opened for us.—HELEN KELLER

MIDNIGHT AND DAWN

We are often creatures of habit, and most of us, from an early age, develop a pattern to our days that works for us. You may not be able to indulge your internal clock—if you are a night owl, for instance, your work may not accommodate the fact that you'd be more comfortable sleeping until noon each day. Still, you find yourself slipping into your natural rhythm when time and life permit: over the weekend, on vacation.

I believe that identifying your internal rhythms and honoring those rhythms is a way of honoring your essence. To live in a constant tug-of-war with your natural cycles is exhausting and ultimately unproductive. And while there are times that we all must work against the clock—internal and external—I encourage you to find a way to allow your life to flow in rhythm with your own cycles.

When you are moving in a state of grace with your essence—with your natural rhythms and patterns—you will unlock creativity, unleash the power and passion of your mind, and free up energy otherwise spent in the constant struggle against the powerful reality of your own unique rhythm.

Identify your personal, internal rhythm. Answer these questions for yourself, and spend time focusing on ways, large and small, that you can best honor your cycles.

- If I could set my own sleep schedule, when would I arise and go to sleep?
- I do my best work between the hours of _____.
- One way I work against my rhythms is _____.
- One way I could work with my rhythms is to _____.

....

DECEMBER 21

A man can't ride your back unless it's bent.—REV. MARTIN LUTHER KING JR.

SURFACING

We all know someone who seems stuck somewhere below the surface, emotionally. Such a person ascribes their behavior to benign or malevolent forces outside of their control. Buffeted by fate or other people or the whims of the world, the un-surfaced person can feel like a loose cannon at times, aimlessly taking aim and firing. You watch yourself around such a person, aware that you may be the next target, although the loose cannon is unlikely to ever acknowledge that the shots fired were meant to harm.

What do you do about someone who will not take responsibility for the ways in which she or he impacts upon you? How do you handle a loose cannon, other than by ducking and dodging?

I recommend modeling: the act of going about your life consciously, focused on remaining surfaced yourself. There is a limited amount you can do to change another, but the possibilities remain endless when it comes to changing yourself. Take control, take responsibility—for yourself. Recognize that the old adage about leading a horse to water is ultimately true, and that your work is not about others; it is about you. Whether the other chooses to follow your path is out of your hands, but if you allow another's behavior to determine which path you take, you are allowing yourself to be pulled under the surface, too.

■ **A CONSCIOUS LIVING PRACTICE FOR TODAY** ■

Look at your circle of friends and family and identify someone who you have thought pulls you under the surface at times, encouraging unconscious living. For today, focus on how you participate with this person in living life under the surface.

- The person I'm thinking of is _____.
- A recent example of un-surfacing is _____.
- I contributed to this un-surfacing by _____.
- The next time such a thing occurs I will _____.

···

DECEMBER 22

There is a time for departure even
when there is no certain place to go.—TENNESSEE WILLIAMS

MASKS

When messages from our deepest selves are ignored, relationships suffer, becoming entanglements of lost souls wearing masks rather than dances of whole beings adorned in their naked truth. Many of us spend our lives struggling to keep secret the shame that often feels as if it runs in the river of our blood. In your journey of conscious living, you focus on uncovering, unfolding. The goal is to accept all of yourself that you see—and to see more and more over time. Your starting point is your commitment to revealing yourself to yourself. You are your only audience. Only you know when you come to love yourself.

■ A CONSCIOUS LIVING PRACTICE FOR TODAY ■

Take three slow, deep, conscious breaths. Visualize a conscious breath as one that fills every corner of your awareness, expanding and cleansing your lungs and your belly, replacing the unconscious breathing that has always sustained you, but nothing more. While you breathe, focus your mind on an intention: loving and accepting yourself completely. Simply breathe fully in and fully out—and while you breathe, imagine the breath filling you with acceptance for everything you are, everything you feel, everything you do. *This* is conscious breathing, and in a breath, you are beginning your journey toward a conscious life.

....

DECEMBER 23

All men should strive to learn before they die
What they are running from, and to, and why.—JAMES THURBER

FOSTERING CREATIVITY

It's to everyone's advantage to foster creativity in the world. Creativity is the unsung hero in every leap forward you make, whether it's a technological breakthrough or finding a new way to appreciate your partner. Creativity requires commitment, and it also requires learning to nurture it. Cultivate a habit of not bashing creative ideas, no matter how ridiculous, unthinkable, or impossible they appear on the surface. Let your mind go a little wild every day. Like the queen in *Alice in Wonderland,* try to think "six impossible things before breakfast."

Make a commitment to creativity today by devoting ten minutes to it. Sometime today, spend ten uninterrupted minutes generating creative ideas in an area you select. Choose your career or your family or any other area of living. Focus on it with the intention of generating creative new ideas that relate to it. Surprise yourself . . . let go and let your wild mind take over. Maybe none of them will turn out to be useful or maybe all of them will. That's not important. What's important is that you followed through on a visible, tangible commitment to creativity.

....

DECEMBER 24

Sit down before fact as a little child, be prepared to give up every preconceived notion, follow humbly wherever and to whatever abyss nature leads, or you shall learn nothing.
—THOMAS HUXLEY

A PLACE IN THE WORLD

As we began this journey, one of the questions that we asked was "Who am I?" Conscious living speaks to the heart of who we are in the universe. It says that we are all equal parts of the whole, and to pretend that we are larger than we are—special cases—is not only a fantasy, but a potentially disastrous one. Conversely, to see ourselves as less significant than we are is equally dangerous.

We must be wary not to embrace any belief that takes us out of oneness with the universe. The moment we do so we render our force-field dense and impermeable.

There is no doubt that the universe is supporting us constantly. From the beginning of life, when we received sustenance through another's body, until today, as you resonate with the universe in a thousand ways, large and small, you are a part of the magical tapestry that is woven of the universe and its inhabitants.

■ A CONSCIOUS LIVING PRACTICE FOR TODAY ■

Close your eyes and breathe deeply. Imagine your world—family, home, work—as a huge tapestry. See yourself as you are, woven into the fabric of this tapestry. When you act outside of your heart—behave in ways that are inconsistent with this universe—you cause an unraveling to begin. Focus on the ways in which you can strengthen the material of your life, of the lives around you.

....

DECEMBER 25
Some are born to sweet delight.—WILLIAM BLAKE

GIVING AND RECEIVING

As humans, we are often creatures of excess. Bigger is better (size *does* count, doesn't it?), more is better, and excess is even better than more. The biggest house, the tallest Christmas tree, the most gifts under the tree; you may find yourself at times in a battle with the universe, one of your own making, to prove that in your excess you are more generous, more successful—and more immortal. Surround yourself with things and you stave off mortality; this is how the thinking seems to unfold. It is as if death will be unable to find you if you are hidden beneath a layer of material coverings.

Today, on the day that many celebrate the birth of Christ, on a day that has become a pageant of giving and receiving, take a few moments to consider what is real. If you stripped down your life to what is most important, most real, what would be left? Relationship. Not houses. Not cars. Not those ribboned gifts under the tree. People would be left.

Knowing this, celebrate your relationships today: their birth, their existence, their importance in your life.

■ **A CONSCIOUS LIVING PRACTICE FOR TODAY** ■

For today, you are going to simplify your celebration.

The most important gifts in my life are _____.

Tell your loved ones what they mean to you today. Celebrate the joyful, hopeful essence of human relationship; honor it by giving voice to how you feel.

....

DECEMBER 26
Every time history repeats itself, the price goes up.—ANONYMOUS

LISTENING TO ERROR MESSAGES

Laura writes: If you use a computer and it's on a certain operating system, you've probably seen a message that flashes ominously on the screen; it says something like this: *Fatal Exception! Error! Fault in Module 12345678! Warning!* Even at the best of moments, it is a dire-sounding alert that something has misfired inside of the brain of the computer. At the worst of times, it can seem as if the computer is somehow aware that the world is coming to an end. Fatal exception, indeed. From personal experience, I attest to the fact that if one ignores the warnings, the consequences (lost files, and worse) can be severe.

Like computers, your own body offers you the same sorts of warnings, although it is up to you to read and interpret the warnings, to pay them heed. When you are on dangerous ground, your body flashes error messages, different for each of you, but easily understood if you just listen. Perhaps you feel a queasiness in your belly, or tension in your neck or shoulders. Perhaps your breath becomes short or your voice changes in pitch. Maybe you experience all of these things in a massive, call-out-the-national-guard warning from your body.

A key part of living consciously is learning to honor the messages your body is sending to you. You must become familiar with these messages—what they are—and you must give yourself the time to stop, to listen, to give yourself the respect you deserve. Time is respect.

■ A CONSCIOUS LIVING PRACTICE FOR TODAY ■

Think of a recent time when things were not going as you wished in your life. After you've read this paragraph, close your eyes and take yourself back to this time and relive how you knew that you were not in synchronicity with your wishes. What physical "error messages" did you give yourself? Did you heed them? If not, why? Make a commitment to yourself to honor yourself by listening closely and respectfully to the messages that you are sending to yourself.

....

DECEMBER 27

In three words I can sum up everything I've learned about life: It goes on.
—ROBERT FROST

PERSPECTIVE

A key learning to take with you on the journey of conscious living is a sense of perspective, a recognition that you must pick your battles, recognize that there *are* some small things in life, and know that there are times when letting go is the greatest gift you can give yourself, whether you are letting go of a feeling, an object, or a person. It's all a question of perspective, of learning to be able to take a step back from your life and see what is important and what is less so. It can be difficult to do this in the thick of things, but it is a skill well worth cultivating.

The essential element in gaining perspective is keeping an eye on yourself, knowing who you are and where you are heading. If you are with yourself, living in a state of integrity—in which you are engaged in an ongoing dialogue with yourself about who you are and what is true for you—perspective will be a natural outgrowth, because things will fall away that do not flow with who you are. The key is to be ever-vigilant in knowing yourself and honoring yourself, and, when you begin to receive the telltale signs from yourself that you are slipping out of integrity, to stop, to listen, to make corrections in a gentle, self-accepting way, to bring yourself back to the state of integrity.

■ A CONSCIOUS LIVING PRACTICE FOR TODAY ■

When you feel the signs from your body that tell you that you are slipping out of a state of integrity, stop what you are doing. Practice now; breathe deeply and slowly and repeat this affirmation aloud: *I commit to being open to hearing the messages from myself about who I am and what it is that I want in my life.*

....

DECEMBER 28

The great cathedral space which was childhood . . . —VIRGINIA WOOLF

ROCK COLLECTIONS

Laura writes: Each of my three sons has gone through a stage of collecting rocks. They are small, plain, garden-variety rocks that are gathered from the yard, the woods, the edges of the roadway running in front of our house. I never collected rocks, so when my oldest son began this stage, I didn't recognize the preciousness of the rocks, which looked to me like ordinary, dirt-covered stones. I learned otherwise when I made the mistake of throwing out a motley collection of the little beige rocks.

With tears in his eyes, my oldest son, Christopher, sat me down when he was four. "Call the police. I have some bad news," he said solemnly. "Someone robbed our house." I looked at him askance, eyebrows raised. "They stoled my rock collection," he said. Fortunately, I recognized the gravity of the situation; had I not been watching his face, I might have chuckled. I suggested Christopher look in his room, and while he was upstairs, I quickly dug the rocks from the trashcan and called to him that I'd found them (I couldn't bear to admit that I'd thrown them away. It suddenly seemed like an outrageous sin). He ran downstairs happily and sat with me, pointing out the special features of each pebble, fifteen or twenty in all. I'd never noticed the many varying shades, the different surface textures, the exquisite variations in size and shape.

Sometimes it takes a child's eyes—or the eyes of someone who hasn't forgotten to see the world with the freshness and leaning toward the precious that a child possesses—to really see what surrounds you. I often wonder, now, what I might be missing around me—and although my house sometimes seems overrun with rocks, I haven't thrown out a pebble in years.

What things of beauty aren't you seeing in your world?

■ A CONSCIOUS LIVING PRACTICE FOR TODAY ■

Today, take five or ten minutes, outside if possible, and free your mind of the limits of seeing through an adult's eyes. Imagine that you are a child again, or someone new to the earth—look at the trees, the plants, the flowers, the earth, the sky . . . and yes, the rocks—with an eye for their beauty. Spend time seeing and feeling the different sizes, shapes, textures, and colors of all that surrounds you. What can you take from this in terms of your own size, your own shape, the texture and color of your life?

DECEMBER 29

Hope is itself a species of happiness, and, perhaps, the chief happiness which this world affords.—SAMUEL JOHNSON

HOPE AND RESOLUTION

You are nearing the end of this year's journey of conscious living—but the end of this year only signals the beginning of another year. In each ending there is, of course, a new beginning. What you make of endings—whether you focus on loss and the sadness of letting go, or whether you look ahead to the possibility that change creates—says much about the way you live your life.

As you think back on this year of learning, knowing, celebrating, look ahead to the new year and to the ways in which you want to integrate the work (and play!) you have done this year into your life in a more permanent manner. Take stock, as many do at year's end, but do it differently; instead of looking for the negative, for that which you have failed to achieve, look for the positive, toward that which you wish to make a part of your life. Conscious learning, conscious love, conscious living—these are the touchstones of my own life, and they serve as reminders to me, daily and as I look back over the year and plan for the new, of what is essential for me. It is my hope that you, too, will continue to find ways to seek, to give, to receive. I wish you consciousness, in all ways, in all seasons, of your life.

■ A CONSCIOUS LIVING PRACTICE FOR TODAY ■

As you near year's end, make a New Year's resolution, but make it grand, make it life-changing and life-affirming. Try beginning with this "thought starter," and then let yourself soar with possibility: *In the next year, what I most want in my life is . . .*

DECEMBER 30

Living is a form of not being sure, not knowing what next or how.
The moment you know how, you begin to die a little.
The artist never entirely knows. We guess. We may be wrong,
but we take leap after leap in the dark.—AGNES DE MILLE

A VERY SPECIAL BIRTHDAY

Although you may join the rest of the world in celebrating New Year's Eve tomorrow, you are also entitled to celebrate a very special birthday. Tomorrow marks a year of focus on living consciously! What a remarkable achievement! Your yearlong commitment to conscious living has brought you through many rich experiences to where you stand right now. Regardless of whether it has been predominantly pleasurable or painful, this special year has been one in which you have done something few people do. Pause to appreciate yourself for what you've done.

Standing in a clear space of heartful appreciation—for where you are and where you've been—look forward now to where you want to go next. What heartsong hums quietly in you, waiting to be brought to full voice? What grand vision inspires you? What will call forth the excellence that will make the next year, and the next and next, a journey of ultimate fulfillment?

These questions of the heart, the mind, and the spirit will be answered one breath at a time, choice by conscious choice. They will be answered as they have been by your fellow travelers on the path of conscious living for thousands of years: by opening up to the power of consciousness and love, the glorious flowers of the human heart and mind, and by committing to care those living treasures forward into the future.

■ A CONSCIOUS LIVING PRACTICE FOR TODAY ■

The work you have done during this past year marks a birth within yourself. It is time to celebrate, and time to give something to yourself to mark this work and this journey. Today, focus on something—material or not—that you can give yourself to celebrate the journey you began a year ago. Some ideas:

- A trip (short or long) to somewhere peaceful and centering.
- A class you've been wanting to take (perhaps a creativity class).
- A book you've wanted to read—and the time to read it.
- A piece of jewelry or article of clothing that represents your journey.
- A piece of artwork that captures the conscious path you have chosen.

....

DECEMBER 31

No person was ever honoured for what he received.
Honour has been the reward for what he gave.—CALVIN COOLIDGE

A TIME FOR HONORING

As your year of living consciously draws toward a close, you are also in a gift-giving time of the year. Be sure you give yourself the gift of taking time out for honoring. Honor yourself for having the courage and commitment to spend a year of your life in a quest for conscious living. Honor all your feelings that have emerged as this year progressed. Honor all the people who have supported you throughout your life. A chance meeting with a person, or the encounter of a certain book at a certain time, may have enabled you on your journey of conscious living.

To pass time in line at a grocery store in 1968, I picked off the rack a paperback about yoga, spontaneously opening it to a section on breathing exercises. That night I tried some of the stretching and breathing practices, making the discovery that they felt delicious to my out-of-shape body. Within a year I'd lost weight, stopped smoking, and put my new learnings to work in my therapy practice. Now I'm a contributor to the field of body-centered psychotherapy and the author of a book entirely about breathing! A magical lifepath—all from a moment's decision in a supermarket.

■ A CONSCIOUS LIVING PRACTICE FOR TODAY ■

Pause now to honor the people and experiences that have influenced you on your journey of living consciously. Send them a silent "thank-you" through the ethers, even if they are long gone. Appreciate them for the blessings they have given you, and bless them in turn on their journey.